Physician's Guide

to Better Medical Decision Making

by Thomas Falasca

About the Author

Dr. Thomas Falasca is an American physician, medical school professor, and medical writer. In addition to medicine, he has degrees in psychology as well as in logic and the philosophy of science. He is board certified in anesthesiology and interventional pain medicine, and has spoken at numerous national and international medical meetings.

Dr. Falasca has long been on the faculty of LECOM Medical School where he has been recipient of the school's Distinguished Teaching Award. At LECOM, he has engaged in classroom lecturing and clinical teaching. He has special experience leading small groups in problem-based learning, applying better medical decision making to clinical cases.

In addition to editing "Evidence-Based Practice Guidelines for Interventional Techniques in the Management of Chronic Spinal Pain," and authoring numerous medical articles, Dr. Falasca has served on the editorial review board for the journal *Pain Physician* and is the content author of the public health and medical information web site *ErieCountyMedicalSociety.org*.

He has served as Secretary of the American Society of Interventional Pain Physicians, as President of the Erie County Medical Society, and on numerous committees of the Pennsylvania Medical Society. He has been recipient of the Distinguished Service Award of the Erie County Medical Society.

Dr. Falasca writes, produces, and is spokesperson for a television series of public service health and medical announcements on ABC affiliate WJET-TV. He produced and hosted the television program *Focus on Erie Medicine* from 1994 until 2011. Finally, he has been a guest on NPR's *The Connection* and has been interviewed by *Time Magazine's* Daniel Eisenberg.

He volunteers with the non-profit Cochrane Collaboration, which produces critical systematic reviews of medical and scientific studies, and with the St. Paul Neighborhood Clinic, which provides free medical services to the disadvantaged.

Dr. Falasca lives in Erie, Pennsylvania and Bergamo, Italy.

Table of Contents

Introduction

Section 1 – Visual Misperceptions

Section 2 – Psychological Biases

Section 3 – Logical Fallacies

Section 4 – Innumeracy

Section 5 – Using Medical Tests

Section 6 – Medical Studies

Section 7 – Evaluating Medications

Conclusion

Further Reading

References

Introduction

Life is short, medicine is long, opportunity fleeting, experience treacherous, judgment difficult. – Hippocrates (460 BC – 370 BC)

Introduction

A book to assist in making better medical decisions is long overdue. A plethora of information in every medical specialty and subspecialty overwhelms physicians daily. However, they find little guiding them to appraise the accuracy of the information or to apply the information appropriately. This book substantially helps fill that vacuum.

Examples of poor medical decision making fill the book, as do plentiful strategic **countermeasures** to identify and avoid such poor medical decisions.

The chapters of *Physician's Guide* comprise several sections that sequentially examine various influences that militate against making sound medical decisions.

The book sections are arranged in an ascending conceptual order with the initial section discussing **perceptions**. Although perceptions are primitive, basic, and seemingly irreducible elements of knowledge, they can be disastrously misleading and are difficult to address.

More complex than perceptions are *judgments under uncertainty*, which can be insidiously perverted by systematic errors known as cognitive **biases**. Biases are not lapses of intelligence or ethics, but are foreseeable human errors made under specific circumstances that the book describes.

When judgments are accumulated and manipulated to draw conclusions, they present the possibility for further errors, called **logical fallacies**. However, since logical fallacies occur at the awareness level, they are more readily addressable than cognitive biases or faulty perceptions.

Numbers, on the other hand, present a special case. First, innumeracy, the limited ability to manipulate numbers, is more socially acceptable than irrationality, the limited ability to manipulate judgments. Second, numbers and statistics frequently receive hasty acceptance under the aura of accuracy. For these reasons, the book introduces concepts and techniques to help clarify numbers and statistics for use in clinical judgment.

Numbers figure prominently in the interpretation of **medical tests**. These tests are optimistically seen as always providing unequivocal, "yes-or-no" answers. However, this sanguine belief is unjustified. Consequently, it is necessary to know to what degree and when medical tests are supportive, when they are disconfirmatory, and when they are inconclusive.

Medical research studies are powerful in that they guide future medical practice. Nevertheless, such studies are easily and frequently flawed, manipulated, and misinterpreted. Fortunately, criteria and tools are available with which to critically evaluate the quality of medical research studies.

The book concludes with a discussion of **medications**. The fact that a medication has been approved for marketing is less informative about its safety and effectiveness than is often thought. Better medical decision making about medication use is necessary in order to employ medications safely and effectively.

The abovementioned book sections are filled with examples from many fields of medicine illustrating the making of poor medical decisions. Moreover, the sections offer powerful countermeasures to avoid such decision-making errors.

Moving forward, the author wishes you an enlightening journey through this oft-neglected area of medicine and a satisfying and fruitful application of better medical decision making to the problems of diagnosis and treatment.

Thomas Falasca
Bergamo, Lombardy, Italy

Visual Perceptions

Chapter 1: Inattention Blindness

Visual Misperceptions

Visual misperceptions undermine confidence in our most reliable knowledge. If concrete visual perceptions can be misleading, how much more misleading can be abstract judgments?

Visual misperceptions highlight this chapter, **inattention blindness**, and the next, **change blindness**.

The present chapter's examination of inattention blindness includes its definition, experimental evidence of its existence, common examples, its destructive influence on medical practice, and medical countermeasures against it.

Inattention Blindness

Inattention blindness is a lack of perception of an unexpected but salient object or event by a subject occupied by other tasks. Inattention blindness is a systematic phenomenon recurring predictably in certain circumstances.

Inattention blindness is perhaps poorly named. The word "inattention" can be construed as pejorative and judgmental. However, the phenomenon is a systematic shortcoming of perception rather than an individual's intellectual or motivational failure. The blindness is substantially related to increased attention being directed to another aspect of the situation. "Inattention blindness" may be more accurately termed "focused attention blindness."

Common Examples – Inattention Blindness

Some common and tragic examples of inattention blindness occur with **accidents involving cars and motorcycles**. The most frequent accident configuration is the motorcycle proceeding straight when the automobile makes a left turn in front of the oncoming motorcycle (Hurt 1981, p. 46). In an alarming number of such accidents, the car driver says that he did not see the motorcycle while the motorcyclist contends the auto driver was "looking right at me." The problem is often that the automobile driver was attending to oncoming traffic looking for a car or truck, but not expecting a motorcycle.

Nevertheless, the results of inattention blindness are not always tragic; sometimes they are downright entertaining. **Magic tricks rely heavily on**

engineered inattention blindness termed variously by magicians as "misdirection" and "attention management." The maneuvers of many magic tricks are executed at a normal pace in plain sight, but are simply not perceived by the audience (Macknik 2012, p. 67).

Peter Vishton reports that one of Harry Blackstone's most famous tricks was a physically simple feat that relied on masterful misdirection. Blackstone always wore a black tuxedo and a large black cape. In one trick, he made a goat seemingly appear magically on stage. In reality, he carried the goat under one arm under the cape and flourished a white handkerchief with the other hand. When he had misdirected the audience, he simply set the goat down and *voila* (Vishton 2011)!

The heavy reliance on misdirection in magic is the main reason for the illusionist's dictum "Never do the same trick for the same audience twice." On the second exposure, the audience is less sensitive to the magician's misdirection and will frequently perceive the formerly unnoticed maneuvers effecting the trick (Macknik 2012, pp. 136-138).

Simons-Chabris Experiments – Inattention Blindness

Simons and Chabris published an experiment in 1999 in which they assembled a white-shirted team of three members and a black-shirted team of three members passing around a basketball. Their subjects watched the event on film and were tasked with counting the number of passes of either the white-shirted team or the black-shirted team (Simons and Chabris 1999).

During the one-minute video, a female student completely covered in a **gorilla suit crossed the screen and remained on camera for nine seconds**. At one point, she even stopped in the middle of the visual field, faced the camera, and thumped her chest. Nevertheless, about half of the subjects reported not seeing the gorilla (Simons and Chabris 1999) (See Picture 1.1).

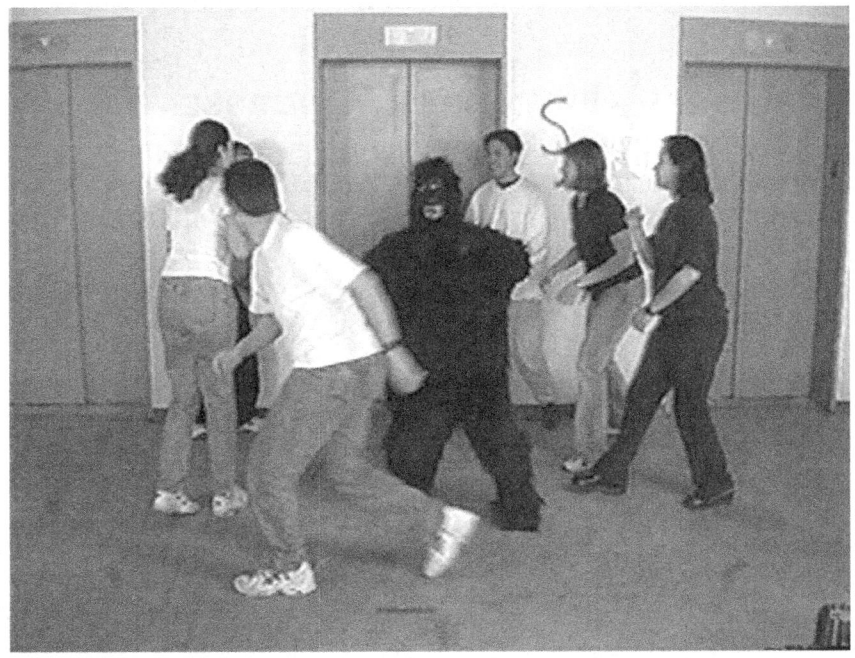

Picture 1.1. Provided by Daniel Simons. To see the video, visit www.dansimons.com or www.theinvisiblegorilla.com.

Finally, the subjects were shown the video again, with the specific instruction to watch for the gorilla. This time some became adamant, stating that the gorilla was not in the video that they first saw and accusing the experimenters of switching the video (Chabris and Simons 2012, p. 7). The video can be viewed at http://www.theinvisiblegorilla.com/videos.html.

Impressively, Daniel Memmert of Heidelberg University repeated the gorilla experiment using an eye tracking device and found that the subjects who failed to notice the gorilla had spent, on average, a full second looking directly at it (Memmert 2006).

The experiment has been repeated many times, under different conditions, with diverse audiences, in many countries, but the results remain unchanged.

Transport for London, the government transit agency for the city, recreated on YouTube a version of the experiment featuring a moonwalking bear. The agency did this as a safety measure to urge awareness to motorists of cyclists on London streets (Transport for London, 2008).

Medical Application - Inattention Blindness

Drew Experiment – Inattention Blindness

The unperceived intrusion of a gorilla into a basketball game may seem remote from medical practice, but Drew and colleagues proved otherwise. These researchers published an experiment in which they assembled 24 radiologists, 15 of whom were expert examiners from the American Board of Radiology (ABR), convened at an ABR meeting in Louisville, Kentucky.

The experimenters asked the radiologists to take three minutes to scroll freely through each of five chest CTs searching for nodules; meanwhile, the experimenters tracked the radiologists' eye positions. The CTs contained an average of 10 nodules and the researchers instructed the radiologists to click on each nodule location with a computer mouse. In the final trial, the researchers inserted a gorilla with a white outline into the area of the lung parenchyma near a lung nodule such that both were clearly visible when the gorilla was at maximum opacity. The gorilla outline measured 29 x 50 mm and faded into and out of visibility over five 2-mm-thick image slices. In total, the gorilla appeared in 239 such slices.

Twenty of the 24 radiologists failed to report seeing the gorilla, although all could see it when they were asked post-experiment to report anything unusual in the slices containing the gorilla (Drew 2013) (See Picture 1.2).

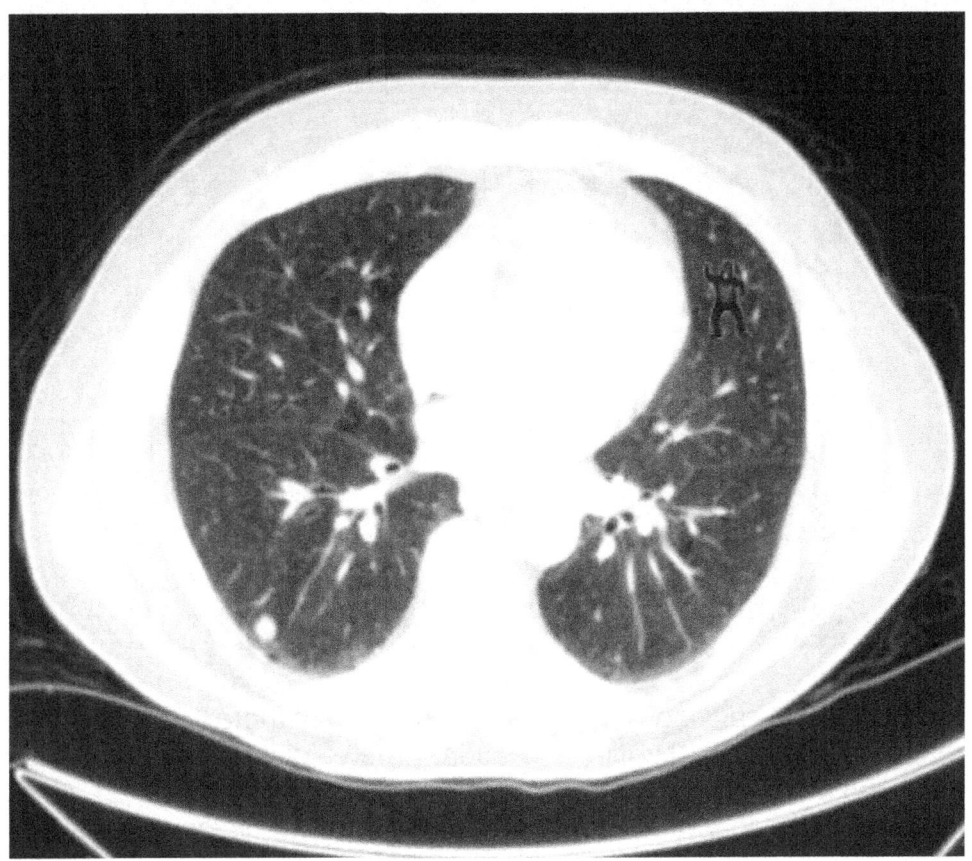

Picture 1.2. Note gorilla upper right of image (left anterior lung field). From Drew 2013, *The Invisible Gorilla Strikes Again*: Sustained Inattentional Blindness in Expert Observers. *Psychological Science, 24*(9), 1848-1853.

Lum Experiment – Inattention Blindness

Lum and colleagues describe the case of a 43 year-old woman admitted through the emergency department with a hematocrit of 7% after three days of profuse vaginal bleeding. The emergency physicians inserted an endotracheal tube, placed a femoral central venous catheter, administered five liters of normal saline and eight units of packed red blood cells, and admitted her to the intensive care unit (ICU). The patient developed pulmonary edema and then pulmonary emboli. During this ordeal, she had three chest x-rays, and a chest CT.

Since she was a poor candidate for anticoagulation, she was scheduled for placement of an inferior vena cava filter. During that procedure, a retained guidewire from the femoral venous catheter insertion was incidentally noted and removed. Retrospectively, the guidewire was clearly visible in the vena cava on the chest CT and all three of the chest x-rays (Lum 2005) (See Picture 1.3).

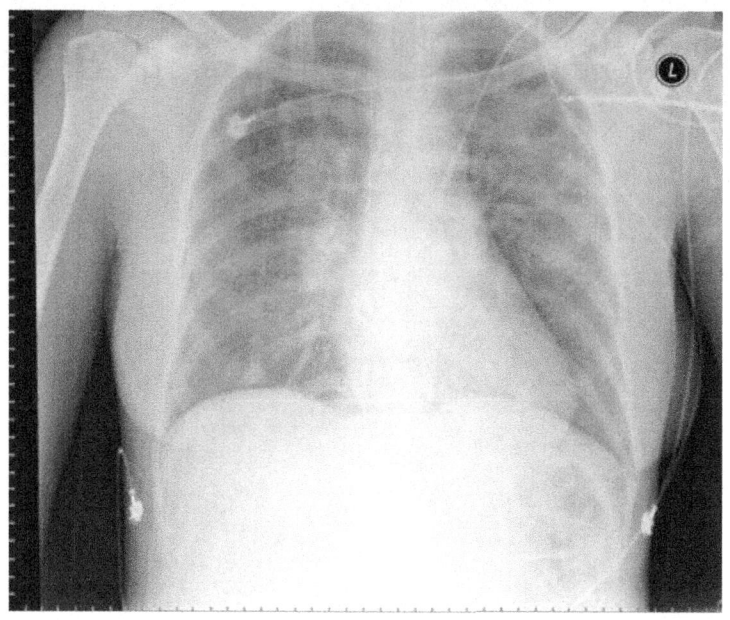

Picture 1.3. Chest X-ray showing guidewire in the right thorax (left side of picture). From Lum 2005, "Profiles in Patient Safety: Misplaced Femoral Line Guidewire and Multiple Failures to Detect the Foreign Body on Chest Radiography" in the *Journal of Academic Emergency Medicine*, June 2008.

It seems incomprehensible that **numerous radiologists, intensivists, and emergency physicians, reading three x-rays and a CT, missed the guidewire.** However, it is more understandable in the context that the physicians were looking for endotracheal tube placement, pulmonary edema, and pulmonary embolism; they were not looking for a retained guidewire. Thus, they succumbed to inattention blindness.

Potchen Experiment – Inattention Blindness

Potchen's 2006 study involved over 100 board certified radiologists. He presented them with 60 chest x-rays, some of which were duplicates. One of the x-rays was of a patient missing a left clavicle. **Over 60% of the radiologists overlooked the missing clavicle** (Groopman 2010, p. 179; Potchen 2006).

Impact of Inattention Blindness

Inattention blindness is characteristically insidious for two reasons:

First, in this blindness, one dangerous situation preempts the perceptual process from another dangerous situation, a situation that may be less frequent, less proximate, or less salient ... but still dangerous! Inattention blindness suggests that the number of parameters to which full attention can be given is limited. This makes countermeasures difficult. Motorists cannot ignore trucks, buses, and cars to attend to motorcycles. Physicians cannot ignore endotracheal tube placement, pulmonary edema, or pulmonary embolism, in a situation especially conducive to these problems, in order to attend to foreign bodies.

Second, perceptions seem so primitive, so simple, and so rooted in reality that subjects fail to question their validity, even though they may question the validity of their own "abstract" evaluations and judgments. This sets up dangerous *inattention-blindness blindness*.

Clinical Practice and Inattention Blindness

In clinical experience, it seems natural to "cut to the chase" and go directly to the most obvious problem. This strategy can be an efficient heuristic, but it also invites inattention blindness. Further, since the strategy often escapes consequences, it invites the overconfidence bias (Chapter 5). Finally, the strategy may be compounded by the *search satisfaction bias* (Chapter 13).

Countermeasures to Inattention Blindness

To begin, it is important to reiterate that phenomena such as inattention blindness are systematic failures of the perception and decision-making processes. As such, they are better dealt with on a systemic basis, than on an individual basis. It is more effective to restructure the environments conducive to these failures than to berate the involved individuals for intellectual or motivational inadequacies.

Countermeasures– Alteration of Configuration

One suggestion that has been offered to the motorcycle "invisibility" problem is an **alteration of configuration**.

Since automobile drivers are looking for an automobile, not a motorcycle, perhaps subtle cues could be introduced to trigger this automobile alertness, such as fitting *motorcycles* with two headlights spaced as widely as possible to activate cues already associated with automobiles (Chabris and Simons 2012, p. 18).

Alteration of configuration is already being used medically. The history of radiology has documented a progression from plain films to contrast studies, to T-weighting in imaging, to energy-sensitive pixel detectors and color images. All these different configurations help reduce inattention blindness by making different aspects of the image more salient.

Another instance of alteration of configuration used in medicine addresses *cell phone distraction in the operating room (OR)*. Following a few high-profile malpractice cases involving inappropriate OR cell phone use, authorities have proposed remedies. One has been to prohibit all cell phone use in patient care areas of the hospital. Another, more realistic, alteration of configuration has been to require OR personnel to have separate cell phones for personal use and for organization of medical information. The personal phone would not be allowed into the OR suite. The medical information phone would be left with a nurse at the scheduling desk; the nurse would monitor the phone and notify the owner only for urgent matters (Hawryluk 2015).

Countermeasures – Sequential Attention

Since attention to one set of parameters has the effect of blinding subjects to other sets of parameters, a useful tool to combat inattention blindness may be **sequential attention** to the various sets of possible parameters.

An example is the sequence of attention involved in reading electrocardiograms (EKG). It is unfortunate that such sequenced evaluation is taught in medical school but often forgotten in the rush of clinical events.

Another example is the sequence of attention encouraged by the various data entry forms now being used for history and physical examination. Of course, it is possible to subvert the purpose of these forms by mechanically checking answers or entering stock responses. Perhaps electronic data records can be designed to reject such maneuvers that subvert the forms' purpose.

A final example of sequence of attention is the variation in any given radiographic or imaging study indicated above. Varying the views, contrast modalities, and energy levels brings sequential attention to different aspects of the study. Thus, altering these parameters both alters configuration and facilitates sequential attention to various aspects of the task. This dimension of the radiologist's practice is sometimes lost on other physicians when they question the value of other studies feeling they have already ordered the *ultimate* study with their MRI request.

Countermeasures – Representative Information

Finally, a countermeasure to unrestrained focus of attention might be the **request for, and submission of, a representative assortment of information**. Here Lum's report of retained guidewire is particularly instructive.

First, a typical complaint of radiologists is that they do not receive sufficient patient information. A radiology request saying nothing more than "pulmonary edema" may be sufficient for billing but may not be sufficient for an effective medical radiological consultation. It seems likely that if the x-ray request had mentioned central venous catheter placement the radiologists would have been checking for a catheter tip and noticed the guide wire.

The information known to the emergency physician but probably lacking to the other doctors in the case was that the patient arrived *in extremis*, was so hypovolemic that no peripheral veins were visible, and that the central venous catheter had to be inserted via the femoral route. The inclusion of such information could well have reduced the influence of inattention blindness.

Second, in this case the failure to supply information might not have been genuine. It is difficult to imagine how the physician placing the catheter did not notice having lost control of the guidewire. Here the guidewire would have been the primary focus of attention not an ancillary focus as encountered by the radiologists reading the x-rays and CT.

Conclusion

This chapter has defined inattention blindness and examined the experimental evidence of its existence. It has explicated inattention blindness's destructive influence on medical practice, and outlined effective medical countermeasures against it. The next chapter will examine inattention blindness's close relative change blindness.

References

Chabris, C. F., & Simons, D. J. (2012). *The invisible gorilla: and other ways our intuitions deceive us*. New York: MJF Books

Drew, T., Võ, M. L. H., & Wolfe, J. M. (2013). The Invisible Gorilla Strikes Again: Sustained Inattentional Blindness in Expert Observers. *Psychological Science, 24*(9), 1848-1853. DOI: 10.1177/0956797613479386

Drew, T., Vo, M., & Wolfe, J. (n.d.). The Invisible Gorilla Strikes Again: © The Author(s) 2013 ... Retrieved April 26, 2017, from http://www.bing.com/cr?IG=565C7E6833A7421790C8C574DAC430EA&CID=1B A56AAB27E861DC15E460DB267860A0&rd=1&h=5eb09o0VmWyOX2GXiRQO6 Wr2_Ln3LqU8kEdTBswykA&v=1&r=http%3a%2f%2fsearch.bwh.harvard.edu%2fnew%2fpubs%2fDre wVoWolfe13.pdf&p=DevEx,5127.1 Visual Attention Lab, Harvard Medical School, and Brigham and Women's Hospital, Boston, Massachusetts

Groopman, J. E. (2010). *How doctors think*. Carlton North, Vic.: Scribe Publications.

Hawryluk, M. (2015, February 2). Is your surgeon focused on you or his smartphone? Texting and surfing can distract from patient care. Bend Bulletin.

Hurt, H. H., Ouellet, J. V., & Thom, D. R. (1981). Motorcycle accident cause factors and identification of countermeasures. Washington, D.C.: National Highway Traffic Safety Administratio

Lum, T. E., Fairbanks, R. J., Pennington, E. C., & Zwemer, F. L. (2005). Profiles in Patient Safety: Misplaced Femoral Line Guidewire and Multiple Failures to Detect the Foreign Body on Chest Radiography. Academic Emergency Medicine,12(7), 658-662. doi:10.1111/j.1553-2712.2005.tb00924.x

Macknik, S. L., Martinez-Conde, S., & Blakeslee, S. (2012). Sleights of mind: what the neuroscience of magic reveals about our brains. London: Profile.

Memmert, D. (2006). The effects of eye movements, age, and expertise on inattentional blindness. Consciousness and Cognition,15(3), 620-627. doi:10.1016/j.concog.2006.01.001

Potchen, E. J. (2006). Measuring Observer Performance in Chest Radiology: Some Experiences. Journal of the American College of Radiology,3(6), 423-432. doi:10.1016/j.jacr.2006.02.020

Simons, D. J., & Chabris, C. F. (1999). Gorillas in Our Midst: Sustained Inattentional Blindness for Dynamic Events. Perception,28(9), 1059-1074. doi:10.1068/p281059

Transport for London. (2008, March 10). Test Your Awareness: Do The Test. Retrieved July 14, 2018, from https://www.youtube.com/watch?v=Ahg6qcgoay4

Vishton, P. M. (2011). Understanding the Secrets of Human Perception. The Teaching Company - The Great Courses. doi:10.1037/e527652012-001

Further Reading

Chabris, C. F., & Simons, D. J. (2012). *The invisible gorilla: and other ways our intuitions deceive us*. New York: MJF Books

Drew, T., Võ, M. L. H., & Wolfe, J. M. (2013). The Invisible Gorilla Strikes Again: Sustained Inattentional Blindness in Expert Observers. *Psychological Science, 24*(9), 1848-1853. DOI: 10.1177/0956797613479386

Groopman, J. E. (2010). *How doctors think*. Carlton North, Vic.: Scribe Publications.

Macknik, S. L., Martinez-Conde, S., & Blakeslee, S. (2012). Sleights of mind: what the neuroscience of magic reveals about our brains. London: Profile.

Simons, D. J., & Chabris, C. F. (1999). Gorillas in Our Midst: Sustained Inattentional Blindness for Dynamic Events. Perception,28(9), 1059-1074. doi:10.1068/p281059

Vishton, P. M. (2011). Understanding the Secrets of Human Perception. The Teaching Company - The Great Courses. doi:10.1037/e527652012-001

Chapter 2: Change Blindness

Change Blindness

Change blindness is a lack of perception of change in a visual stimulus from what was in view a few moments ago to what is in view now (Chabris 2012, p. 54).

Common Examples – Change Blindness

A **card trick** described by magician and physicist Alex Stone poignantly exemplifies change blindness. Here, in the pre-trick set-up, the magician removes the *eight of clubs* and *nine of spades* from the deck and places them on top of the deck. Then, in the presence of the audience, he removes the similar looking *nine of clubs* and *eight of spades*, shows them to the audience, and inserts them into the *middle* of the deck. Finally, after a suitable gesture or incantation, he claims to have moved them to the *top* of the deck. He turns over the top two cards and, sure enough, there are the *eight of clubs* and *nine of spades* (Stone 2012, p. 200). Presto! The only magic word here is *change blindness*!

While the magician maximizes the opportunities for change blindness, the movie director minimizes the opportunities for change blindness.

Movies are seldom shot in real time. More often, a scene is shot over a few days or weeks. One clue to a segment change within a scene is a shift in camera view. Each of these times a scene needs to be reconstructed, a continuity editor verifies that clothing, furniture, and accessories remain the same.

Nevertheless, there are occasional continuity failures. When the camera cuts away, there are three chairs at the table; when it returns, there are four! When the camera cuts away, an actress is wearing a necklace; when it returns, the necklace is gone!

Continuity failures have produced a cult following of devotees dedicated to finding continuity errors in television series such as *Friends* and movies such as *The Godfather*.

A final example of change blindness comes from the reports of physician-author **Arthur Conan Doyle, creator of Sherlock Holmes**. Doyle often said that the inspiration for the observational skills of the storied detective was one of his medical school professors at Edinburgh, surgeon Joseph Bell. Dr. Bell exhibited unusual abilities of observation and challenged his students to do the same.

On one such occasion, Dr. Bell is reported to have stood before his class with an open vial of liquid of intensely bitter taste and offensive smell. He then dipped a finger into the liquid and placed his finger into his mouth. He passed the vial of liquid around the class inviting the aspiring doctors to do the same. The vial made its way around the lecture room leaving behind a trail of grimaced faces. When the vial returned to him, Dr. Bell announced his disappointment in the class. He reprimanded his students that no one had noticed that he had dipped his *index* finger into the vial but had tasted his *middle* finger!

Simons-Levin Experiments – Change Blindness

Levin and Simons published an experiment in 1997 in which they made a 40-second film featuring characters Andrea and Sabrina sitting across a table planning a party. There were seven cuts in which the camera sometimes angled on Andrea, sometimes on Sabrina, and sometimes on both. During the seven cuts, Levin and Simons had placed nine continuity errors.

The experimenters showed this sound video to 10 subjects who were instructed to "pay close attention" but were not forewarned of the changes. Only one of the 10 subjects noted any change after the first viewing. After being cued that changes might involve "objects, body positions, or clothing," the subjects viewed the film a second time. This time they reported an average of only two of the nine changes (Levin and Simons 1997).

Levin and Simons next determined to carry their investigation into the real world. They constructed an experiment in which an actor carrying a map stopped a naive pedestrian ostensibly to ask directions. About 10-15 seconds into the interaction, **two other actors carrying a door stepped between the actor soliciting directions and the naive pedestrian**, the experimental subject. As the door passed, the rearward door carrier, carrying an identical map, switched places with the original direction-seeker.

Of the 15 pedestrian subjects involved, only 7 noticed the change despite obvious differences between the actors in appearance, clothing, and voice (Levin and Simons 1998).

Medical Examples - Change Blindness

In 2010, **dialysis patient Richard Smith** was admitted to the intensive care unit (ICU) at North Shore Medical Center in Miami because of shortness of breath following a dialysis session. The next day he complained of an upset stomach. To inhibit gastric acid production, his physician prescribed an injection of *Pepcid*

™. However, his nurse, Uvo Ologboride misidentified the package and injected the potent neuro-muscular blocker *pancuronium* instead. Mr. Smith went into respiratory arrest and entered a vegetative state, dying a month later.

Of course, change blindness was only the initiating factor here. There were multiple failures. Certainly, to obviate change blindness, the nurse was required to carefully read the package, to read the bottle within the package before drawing up the medication, and to read the bottle again after drawing up the medication. Nurse Ologboride failed to do all of these things.

Another case involving change blindness occurred at a **women's clinic in Birmingham, UK** in October 2006. One woman, who had already been seen at the clinic for her preliminary visits, was scheduled to return for a chemical abortion. On the morning of her scheduled abortion, another patient with the same first name appeared for a first visit.

Only first names were used in the reception area to protect patient privacy. When the first name was called, the new patient responded. None of the personnel noticed that this was not the patient they had seen previously. The new patient, who would never have qualified for a chemical abortion, was shown to a treatment room where nurse Downer administered the abortifacient. The new patient remarked how quickly this all went and left for home.

A little later, the intended patient arrived. Her chart could not be found in either the arriving patient file or the general patient file. It was finally discovered in the file for patients already treated. Only then was the error discovered. Several staff members all missed the substitution.

Again, change blindness was only the initiating factor. Back-up systems to obviate this type error were already in place, but were circumvented. Once the patient was beyond the reception area, her full name and identifying information was to have been confirmed, but it was not.

Finally, a more benign medical instance of change blindness occurs frequently. Plastic surgeons warn, and plastic surgery patients acknowledge, that friends and **acquaintances of plastic surgery patients often fail to notice that anything has changed,** sometimes after even extensive surgery.

Countermeasures to Change Blindness

Unsurprisingly, some of the same countermeasures to inattention blindness are also countermeasures to change blindness.

An **alteration of configuration** countermeasure suggested during the investigation of the above case of Richard Smith, who died after receiving the paralyzing agent pancuronium, was that the pancuronium should never have been in the ICU. While it may be difficult comment on that particular suggestion, it seems obvious that other alterations of configuration may also be possible.

Certainly, infrequently used, potentially lethal drugs as pancuronium can be kept out of proximity to frequently used, relatively innocuous medications as Pepcid^{TM}. Again, if the packaging of pancuronium is similar to that of common innocuous medications, it seems the manufacturer could package them differently or the hospital pharmacy could double package them or alter the packaging to create a more obvious difference.

Sequential attention in change blindness is somewhat different from what it is in inattention blindness. Here it involves *repetitive identification*, as in the nurse being required to check the medication label on opening the package, again on drawing up the medication, and yet again after drawing up the medication.

Sequential attention as a countermeasure to change blindness is useful regarding the patient as well as regarding the medication.

Patient identification is recommended to be by at least two *independent* parameters, such as the patient's statement (not merely confirmation) of name, social security number, phone number, birth date, or patient identification number. This is then verified against the patient's wristband and chart documentation.

Surgical site is marked by the surgeon in advance and verified against the chart and the patient's understanding before the procedure. The marking is by indelible marker to withstand the surgical prep.

A final sequential step is the *surgical "time out,"* in which patient identity and procedure are verified in the operating room (OR) before surgery commences.

These measures all seem like substantial steps; nevertheless, capitulating to the availability bias (Chapter 3) and identifying patients by bed number or room number sets the stage for the operation of change blindness.

Conclusion

This chapter has examined the unreliability of some perceptions especially with application to medicine. Further, it has offered countermeasures to help attenuate the blinding effect.

Finally, the blinding effect provides a valuable lesson and inspires a central question. Perceptions seem so primitive, so simple, and so rooted in reality. If perceptions are unreliable, how much more so are memories, judgments, decisions, and other mental processes?

References

Chabris, C. F., & Simons, D. J. (2012). *The invisible gorilla: and other ways our intuitions deceive us*. New York: MJF Books

Levin, D. T., & Simons, D. J. (1997). Failure to detect changes to attended objects in motion pictures. Psychonomic Bulletin & Review,4(4), 501-506. doi:10.3758/bf03214339

Simons, D. J., & Levin, D. T. (1998). Failure to detect changes to people during a real-world interaction. Psychonomic Bulletin & Review,5(4), 644-649. doi:10.3758/bf03208840

Stone, A. (2012). Fooling Houdini: magicians, mentalists, math geeks, and the hidden powers of the mind. New York: Harper.

Further Reading

Chabris, C. F., & Simons, D. J. (2012). *The invisible gorilla: and other ways our intuitions deceive us*. New York: MJF Books

Psychological Bias

Chapter 3: Definition of Bias and Anchoring Bias

Definition of Bias

Bias, also known as **psychological bias** or **cognitive bias**, is a tendency to think in certain ways that can lead to systematic deviations from a standard of rationality or good judgment (Wikipedia 2017). Biases are systematic errors that recur predictably in certain circumstances (Kahneman 2015, p. 3, Kindle edition).

Biases are *patterns* of behavior assessed from observing the behavior of groups of people. Thus, they are not judgments of the intellectual or character failings of a particular individual. Biased behaviors occur even when subjects are encouraged to be accurate and are rewarded for the correct answers (Tversky and Kahneman 1972 and 1973). They even occur when subjects are forewarned about them (Wilson 1996). Most subjects report being uninfluenced by their biases, while the data show otherwise (Wilson 1996).

Biases have been shown to exert their influence in judicial circumstances, when the experimental subjects were experienced judges making determinations in fictitious legal cases (Englich 2006). Biases have been shown to exert their influence in medical circumstances, when the subjects were examiners from the American Board of Radiology reading routine chest x-rays (Drew 2013).

Finally, biases operate below the level of attention and are poorly addressed by exhortations to "Wake-up," "Pay attention," or "Be more careful!"

Initiating the discussion of the more common biases is the anchoring bias.

Anchoring Bias

Anchoring bias is reliance on a past reference or on one piece of information, often the first piece of information, when making decisions, even when the comparison anchor is completely arbitrary (Shermer 2012).

Common Examples – Anchoring Bias

The world abounds with examples of the anchoring bias. Auto manufacturers quote a high manufacturer's suggested retail price (MSRP) so that purchasers begin with that number in mind and consider anything less a bargain.

Home sellers begin with a "high ball" asking price expecting to lower it so that purchasers feel they are receiving a great home as well as a great bargain.

A 10% off sale for Campbell's soup at a Sioux City, Iowa supermarket provides another interesting example. When a sign that read "Limit of 12 per Customer" accompanied the display, the average customer bought seven cans. When the "limit of 12" sign was removed, the average customer's purchase fell to about half that number (Kahneman 2015, p. 126).

Tversky/Kahneman Experiments – Anchoring Bias

Kahneman and Tversky constructed an experiment in which they rigged a wheel of fortune to stop at either 10 or 65. With their subject in front of them, they would then spin the wheel and ask the subject to write down the number at which the wheel stopped.

They then asked their subject two questions: First, "Is the percentage of African nations among UN members larger or smaller than the number you just wrote?" Second, "What is your best guess of the percentage of African nations in the UN?"

The average estimate of subjects who saw 10 was 25%. The average estimate of those who saw 65 was 45% (Tversky and Kahneman 1974; Kahneman 2015, p. 119).

In another experiment Kahneman and Tversky used as subjects two groups of high school students. They asked each group to estimate within 5 seconds the product of the same eight numbers. But for one group, they presented the numbers as the written sequence "1 x 2 x 3 x 4 x 5 x 6 x 7 x 8" and for the other group, the written sequence "8 x 7 x 6 x 5 x 4 x 3 x 2 x 1." They reasoned that 5 seconds was enough time for subjects to multiply only the first few numbers of the sequence.

The median estimate for the group given the ascending sequence was 512, while the median estimate for the group given the descending sequence was 2,250. The correct answer is 40,320 (Tversky and Kahneman 1974).

Englich/Mussweiler/Strack Experiment – Anchoring Bias

Three German psychologists demonstrated the anchoring bias with an experiment using as subjects 52 recent law graduates at a national postgraduate training program in Speyer, Germany.

The subjects were instructed to assume the role of trial judge in a fictitious shoplifting case involving a woman who had stolen items from a supermarket for the 12th time. The subjects were told to consider the expert opinion of a forensic psychologist, as well as statements by the defendant and a witness.

The role-playing judges were instructed that they would learn the prosecutor's demand for sentencing by rolling a pair of dice. They were not told that the dice of one pair had been loaded so that the dice always showed a one and a two while the other pair had been loaded so that the dice always showed a three and a six.

Results were that the role-playing judges rolling the low-loaded dice gave a mean sentence of 5.28 months probation while those rolling the high-loaded dice gave a mean sentence of 7.81 months probation (Englich, Mussweiler, and Strack 2006).

Another version of the experiment demonstrated similar results. However, in this version, the subjects were not 52 recent law school graduates role-playing judges, but 23 experienced judges and 19 experienced prosecutors at an average age of 42 years and average experience of 11 years (Englich, Mussweiler, and Strack 2006).

Medical Examples of the Anchoring Bias

Certainly, physicians have many occasions to be influenced by the anchoring bias.

- Do physicians treat prehypertension differently if they think first of 120/80 or think first of 140/90?
- Do pharmaceutical companies that manufacture antihypertensive drugs try getting physicians to anchor on lower numbers to initiate treatment?
- Do physicians questioning an evasive or vague patient, sufficiently consider the examples they offer in order to avoid influencing the patient's answer.
- Do surgeons, when presenting patients with a surgical intervention that has infrequent fatal complications and more frequent, minor complications, change the patient's acceptance probability when listing the complications in a descending order of severity or in a descending order of frequency?

In another medical application, physicians have long been advocating for caps on pain and suffering in medical professional liability cases. Physicians have felt that this would lower their professional liability insurance premiums. However, Kahneman warns that having such a cap might establish an anchor. He indicates that the anchor might *lower* the less numerous higher awards to the level of the cap but *raise* the more numerous lower awards to the level of the cap, possibly increasing liability premiums (Kahneman 2015, p. 127).

Countermeasures to the Anchoring Bias

Countermeasures are difficult to implement when the subjects of the bias are unaware of its influence upon them.

One clue to a potential countermeasure is contained in Wilson's finding (Wilson 1996). He and his colleagues determined that the amount of knowledge that subjects have of the target question moderated the effects of the anchoring bias. Perhaps this provides more information on which to anchor thus canceling extreme anchors. In brief, having and considering a great deal of experience and information seems to provide an ameliorating effect on the anchoring bias.

Another possible countermeasure to the anchoring bias may be to revisit decisions intermittently and avoid isolated impulsive decisions. For the physician, this means periodically evaluating an established patient afresh, with new eyes. In this way, anchors that are difficult to eradicate might at least counterbalance one another when encountered on a random schedule.

It is encouraging that anchoring and other biases have been identified. However, much work remains to be done on techniques to reduce their deleterious effects on decision-making.

Conclusion

It is disconcerting to think that the anchoring bias can surreptitiously and significantly change decisions of physicians and patients. At least the bias is known, countermeasures are available, and more measures are likely to emerge as additional information about the bias develops.

References

Drew, T., Vo, M., & Wolfe, J. (n.d.). The Invisible Gorilla Strikes Again: © The Author(s) 2013 ... Retrieved April 26, 2017, from http://www.bing.com/cr?IG=565C7E6833A7421790C8C574DAC430EA&CID=1B A56AAB27E861DC15E460DB267860A0&rd=1&h=5eb09o0VmWyOX2GXiRQO6 Wr2_Ln3LqU8kEdTB-swykA&v=1&r=http%3a%2f%2fsearch.bwh.harvard.edu%2fnew%2fpubs%2fDre wVoWolfe13.pdf&p=DevEx,5127.1

Visual Attention Lab, Harvard Medical School, and Brigham and Women's Hospital, Boston, Massachusetts

Englich, B., Mussweiler, T., & Strack, F. (2006). Playing Dice With Criminal Sentences: The Influence of Irrelevant Anchors on Experts' Judicial Decision Making. Personality and Social Psychology Bulletin,32(2), 188-200. doi:10.1177/0146167205282152

Kahneman, D. (2015). *Thinking, fast and slow*. New York: Farrar, Straus and Giroux.

Shermer, M. (2012). *The believing brain: from ghosts and gods to politics and conspiracies--how we construct beliefs and reinforce them as truths*. New York: St. Martin's Griffin.

Tversky, A., & Kahneman, D. (1974). Judgment under Uncertainty: Heuristics and Biases. *Science, 185*(4157), 1124-1131. doi:10.1126/science.185.4157.1124

Wilson, T. D., Houston, C. E., Etling, K. M., & Brekke, N. (1996). A new look at anchoring effects: Basic anchoring and its antecedents. Journal of Experimental Psychology: General,125(4), 387-402. doi:10.1037//0096-3445.125.4.387

Further Reading

Kahneman, D. (2015). *Thinking, fast and slow*. New York: Farrar, Straus and Giroux.

Shermer, Michael. (2012). The Believing Brain: From Ghosts and Gods to Politics and Conspiracies---How We Construct Beliefs and Reinforce Them as Truths. Henry Holt and Co.. Kindle Edition.

Tversky, A., & Kahneman, D. (1974). Judgment under Uncertainty: Heuristics and Biases. *Science, 185*(4157), 1124-1131. doi:10.1126/science.185.4157.1124

Chapter 4: Availability and Confirmatory Biases

Availability and Confirmatory Biases

Probably the two cognitive biases most frequently affecting, or more accurately "mal-affecting," medical decision making are the **availability bias** and the **confirmatory bias**, which often appear together. Descriptions of these two biases follow, along with discussions of the experimental evidence for their existence, clinical examples of their role in poor medical decisions, and, finally, strategies for overcoming them.

Availability Bias

Availability bias is a tendency to judge entities that come to mind more readily as also being more probable or more frequent (Crowley, Legowski, Medvedeva, et al 2013). Readiness to come to mind, in turn, can be influenced by the event's drama, its vividness, its recent occurrence, or even its recent conversational mention.

One of the first to describe the availability bias, Daniel Kahneman, classified it as a substitution heuristic because it exchanges one parameter for another. In this case, the *ease* with which an event comes to mind substitutes for the *frequency* or *probability* of the event (Kahneman 2011).

Kahneman also points out that the availability bias affects knowledgeable novices more than true experts and affects those engaged in simultaneous effortful tasks more than those not so engaged (Kahneman 2011). Perhaps a little knowledge is a dangerous thing and multitasking comes with a price.

Common Examples of the Availability Bias

Some of the most compelling examples of the availability bias come from the work of Lichtenstein, Slovic, and Fischhoff (1978) who rigorously compared the frequency of lethal events as perceived by experimental subjects with the actual frequencies of the events at the time of the study. Some of the results were as follows:

- Approximately 80% of the subjects judged accidental death as more likely than death from stroke, although strokes caused almost twice as many deaths as all accidents combined.
- The subjects estimated tornadoes as more frequent killers than asthma,

although asthma caused 20 times as many deaths as tornadoes.
- The experimental subjects judged botulism as causing more deaths than lightning, although deaths from lightning were 52 times more frequent than deaths from botulism.
- The subjects deemed death from accident and from disease to be about equally frequent, although death from disease was 18 times more likely than accidental death.
- Finally, the subjects judged deaths from accidents to be 300 times more frequent than death from diabetes, whereas diabetes-related deaths outnumbered accidental deaths 4 to 1.

Other examples of the availability bias also abound:
- The "sophomore syndrome" affects second year medical students who imagine themselves to have the diseases they study.
- Medical undergraduates endeavoring to read EKGs often overlook the assessment of rate, rhythm, and axis, instead skipping ahead to evaluation of the more available morphology.
- Increased volumes of patients present for evaluation for a specific disease soon after appearance in the news of a celebrity diagnosed with that disease.
- Increased numbers of physicians diagnose the disease when it is in the news.
- The availability bias is evident in the preoccupation of many patients with side effects. Here, patients may tend to judge as more probable the well-defined side effects of therapy than the uncertain and protean consequences of disease (Groopman 2010, p. 246).

The existence of the availability bias supports the need for general internists and family practice physicians in the medical community. These generalist physicians serve to counterbalance the tendency of specialists and subspecialists to think in terms of the more available concepts of their own more narrow disciplines.

Schwarz Experiment – Availability Bias

Norbert Schwarz constructed an intriguing study of the availability bias. He asked his subjects, all West German university students, to rate their assertiveness after first enumerating either 6 or 12 instances in which they believed they had acted assertively. He reasoned that 6 memories of assertive behavior would come to mind more easily than 12 and thus would be more available. Results showed that the students who were required to list 6 instances of assertiveness rated themselves as more assertive than the students who were required to list 12 instances.

Moreover, Schwarz's study was a *crossover* experiment in which Schwarz next asked his subjects to rate their unassertiveness after first enumerating either 6 or 12 instances in which they believed they had acted *unassertively*. The students who were required to list 6 instances of *unassertiveness* rated themselves as more *unassertive* than the students who were required to list 12 instances (Schwarz 1991).

In short, the students who rated themselves *assertive* when that choice was more available also rated themselves as *unassertive* when that choice was more available.

Kahneman and Tversky Experiment – Availability Bias

Kahneman and Tversky constructed an experiment in which they presented 152 subjects with the consonants K, L, N, R, and V. They asked the subjects if they thought the letters occurred more often in the first or third position in words in the English language. Further, they asked the subjects to estimate the relative frequencies with which the letters occupied those positions (Kahneman and Tversky 1973).

Of the 152 subjects, 105 judged the first position to be more frequent for a majority of the letters and they judged the letters to occupy the first position twice as often as they occupied the third position. In fact, all of the five letters occur more frequently in the third position. The subjects were biased in favor of the cognitively more available first position.

Confirmatory Bias

Confirmatory bias, or **confirmation bias**, is the seeking, recognizing, or interpreting of evidence in ways that are partial to existing beliefs, expectations, or hypotheses. Francis Bacon noted confirmatory bias in his 1620 treatise *Novum Organum* (Nickerson 1998).

The confirmatory bias can involve not only the selective seeking, recognizing, or overvaluing of evidence in support of a preconceived idea, but also the selective dismissing, blindness to, or undervaluing of contradictory evidence. The bias is insidious in that it operates below the conscious level and so can be resistant to conscious corrective action.

Darley and Gross Experiment – Confirmatory Bias

Darley and Gross performed a study in 1983 in which they divided their subjects into two groups, each of which was shown the video of a child taking an academic test. Prior to viewing the video, one group was told that the child came from an upper socioeconomic level while the other group was told that the child came from a lower socioeconomic level. No part of the socioeconomic information contained any reference to the child's academic status.

Following the video, both groups were asked to review the child's completed test and rate the child's academic performance with respect to grade level. Although both groups saw the same video and the same completed academic test, those who were told that the child came from a higher socioeconomic status tended to rate the child as performing above grade level. Those who were told that the child came from a lower socioeconomic status tended to rate the child as performing below grade level. Each group cited aspects of the test to support their conclusion (Darley and Gross 1983).

Common Examples of the Confirmatory Bias

The confirmatory bias has been cited in the explanation of numerous phenomena:
- **Conspiracy theories**. Only data supporting the conspiracy gains the attention of the conspiracy believer. Contradictory data do not seem to rise above the believer's awareness threshold.
- **Kennedy-Lincoln relationship**. Soon after the assassination of John F. Kennedy there arose the contention of a mysterious link between the two Presidents based on a number of parallels:
  - Both were shot in the head on a Friday.
  - Both their wives lost children while living in the White House.
  - Both had a Vice-President named Johnson.
  - Kennedy's assassin fled from a warehouse and was caught in a theater; Lincoln's assassin fled from a theater and was caught in a warehouse.
  - Kennedy was elected President in 1960; Lincoln was elected President in 1860.

Of course, here only the parallels come to mind, not the multitudinous aspects in which the two men were completely different.

Toupee fallacy. This interesting fallacy affects people who are convinced that they can always spot a man wearing a toupee. Unfortunately, they reach this conclusion because they are only aware of the instances in which they spot the toupee and unaware of the instances in which they miss it (Novella 2012).

Vaccination phobia. In 1998, London physician Andrew Wakefield published an article in *The Lancet* suggesting a link between the measles-mumps-rubella (MMR) vaccine and autism. This was based on the claims of eight parents that their children began demonstrating the symptoms of autism at about the time of their vaccination. Although Wakefield promoted an association between MMR and autism in press conferences (Chabris, Simons 2010), no causal connection between MMR vaccination and autism was ever demonstrated.

Evidence of no vaccination-autism connection came from a fortuitous event and an alert Japanese psychiatrist, Hideo Honda, who studied a population of 300,000 in Yokohama. Yokohama 's MMR vaccination program began in 1989 but was terminated in 1993 because of an increased frequency of aseptic meningitis suspectedly related to components of the vaccine. Honda and colleagues then studied this population for the years 1989 through 1996. Nevertheless, they found that the autism diagnoses in the area began a steady *increase* rather than a *decrease* after 1993 (Honda 2005).

Further evidence of no vaccination-autism connection came from a study of all Danish children born from January 1991 through December 1998. This study found the frequency of autism to be similar in the vaccinated and unvaccinated kids. Further, it found no temporal clustering of autism cases at any time after vaccination. Impressively, the study involved a nationwide cohort and nearly complete follow-up data (Madsen 2002).

Meanwhile, Wakefield's 1998 paper was found to be fraudulent. *The Lancet* retracted its publication of his paper and Wakefield was struck from the United Kingdom Medical Register and prohibited from practicing medicine in the UK.

Further, Wakefield did not disclose that the eight "sequential" referrals were a group referred by a law firm that had already paid him £75,000. Eventually, he received almost £700,000 in expert legal fees.

Worse, he was found to have acted without ethical approval from an institutional review board. He was deemed to have been responsible for submitting children with autism to unnecessary colonoscopies and lumbar punctures. One of the children suffered 12 bowel punctures during colonoscopy, was in ICU, suffered kidney, liver, and neurological injuries, and received £740,000 in compensation (Goldacre 2010, Kindle locations 3010-3028).

Meanwhile, measles cases increased sharply in recent years, almost entirely among the unvaccinated, according to the US Centers for Disease Control and Prevention. Because of Wakefield's contribution to the increase, *Medscape* rated him as the worst of the worst in 2011 in its "Physicians of the Year: Best and Worst." This title indicated that Wakefield was held in less esteem than other major candidates that year, including the infamous Conrad Murray, convicted in 2011 of involuntary manslaughter in the death of Michael Jackson.

Yet, in one national survey, 29% of those queried agreed that vaccines were responsible for causing autism (Chabris, Simons 2010. P. 183 of 242, location 3130 of 5519.) In March 2015, the Oregon Chiropractic Association invited him to testify in opposition to Senate Bill 442, which would eliminate nonmedical exemptions from Oregon's school immunization law. In April 2015, Wakefield was given two standing ovations by students of Life Chiropractic College West when he told them to oppose Senate Bill 277 that would limit non-medical vaccine exemptions. The respondents to the national survey, the Oregon Chiropractic Association, and the students of Life College all fell victim to the confirmatory bias.

Medical Examples of the Availability and Confirmatory Biases

Anecdotal Examples

Anecdotal medical examples of the availability bias certainly come to mind.

It is widely believed that the lower hemoglobin and hematocrit in women vs. men is fully explained by the occurrence of menses. The less dramatic lower testosterone level in women seems to receive substantially less consideration although it is of considerable significance.

Additionally, it is interesting that cases of a single rare diagnosis occasionally come in groups. Sometimes this phenomenon is explained by the first instance of such a diagnosis "priming" the physician and making the diagnosis more available in his/her mind. Thereupon the physician makes the diagnosis more frequently, at least for a period of time. The "priming" effect seems to have a limited duration.

A final example, this one combining the availability and confirmatory biases is the tendency of reductionism, which seeks to reduce one discipline to another. One often hears the contention that medicine is really just pharmacy or medicine is really just a business. Here medicine is reduced to some available activity and only confirming evidence is sought or considered. If medicine is just pharmacy, then how explain surgery? If medicine is just another business, then how explain physicians' activities in prevention and public health, activities that potentially put them out of business? These disconfirmatory evidences escape consideration.

Case Examples

It is appropriate now to exemplify how the availability and confirmatory biases can impact clinical medical decision making. The cases analyzed here are from among those presented in *Avoiding Errors in General Practice* (Barraclough et al 2013). These examples demonstrate the subtle forms biases can manifest.

Elderly Man with Sinusitis

Case

Alfred was a 74 year-old man who presented to Dr. McDowd reporting a two-week history of fever, sinusitis, loss of appetite, and loss of weight that he attributed to his lower dentures interfering with eating. Dr. McDowd found him afebrile with a clear chest and treated him with amoxicillin.

Eight days later Alfred re-consulted Dr. McDowd with complaints of increased weight loss and continued sinus pain. Dr. McDowd found a temperature of 37.4° C, normal pulse, and normal blood pressure; he changed the amoxicillin to doxycycline.

Three days later Alfred's wife phoned Dr. McDowd that Alfred was not eating and not himself. Dr. McDowd ordered blood tests and sinus x-rays. Alfred presented at the practice the following day and saw McDowd's colleague Dr. Ellsworth, who noted weight loss and sinusitis. Alfred had not had the sinus x-rays done. Dr. Ellsworth prescribed clarithromycin and a nasal decongestant.

The following day Dr. McDowd received the blood test results indicating a CRP of 70 mg/l (reference 0-10 mg/l), an ESR of 64 mm/hr (reference <20 mm/hr), and Hb of 10.9 g/dl (reference 13.5-17.5). Dr. McDowd also reviewed the report of an optometrist indicating that Alfred had intermittent diplopia. Dr. McDowd ordered serum ferritin, B12, folate, and fasting blood glucose.

The following day, Alfred phoned Dr. McDowd that he had no vision in his left eye. Dr. McDowd sent him immediately to the emergency department. There he was found to have impalpable temporal arteries and a history of jaw claudication and bitemporal headache. Alfred was diagnosed with giant cell arteritis and treated with high-dose methylprednisolone, but he never regained the vision in his left eye.

Commentary

Dr. McDowd was overtaken by the availability and confirmatory biases. He immediately fixed upon the available diagnosis of sinusitis submitted by the patient. However, his confirmatory evidence was no more than a clear chest on auscultation. Moreover, the most relevant signs and symptoms are 1) purulent nasal secretion, 2) abnormal sinus trans-illumination, 3) maxillary toothache, 4) poor response to nasal decongestants, and 5) history of colored nasal discharge. When all five are present, the odds of sinusitis increase sharply. When none are present, sinusitis is ruled out (Williams and Simel pp. 598). Nevertheless, McDowd appears not to have considered (or at least, not to have documented) any of these signs and symptoms.

The disconfirming evidence of afebrile or minimally febrile state seems to have been overlooked entirely.

Eight days later, when the patient worsened, McDowd changed the antibiotic but did not entertain reconsidering the diagnosis.

Three days later, when the patient continued to deteriorate, Dr. Ellsworth also changed the antibiotic without reconsidering the diagnosis. It is interesting that this confirmatory bias continued even when a new physician saw the patient. Dr. Groopman calls this "diagnosis momentum" (Groopman 2008).

The next day, McDowd received lab results of markedly elevated CRP and ESR along with markedly reduced Hb. However, he did not even consider the abnormal CRP and ESR. Moreover, he sought to relate the reduced Hb to a completely new diagnosis rather than considering if it could be related to the patient's original complaints.

The following day, when the patient complained of vision loss in the left eye, McDowd sent him to the emergency department, where the diagnosis was made.

In this case, the availability bias and the confirmatory bias cost the patient the vision in his left eye.

Injury from Playing Badminton

Case

Paul was a 45 year-old male who felt a snap in his right calf while playing badminton. Three days later, he consulted Dr. du Vivier who noted right calf swelling and intact Achilles tendon, and diagnosed muscle strain.
Symptoms failed to improve and 3 weeks later Paul consulted Dr. Prasad, who concurred with the muscle strain diagnosis and prescribed exercises and naproxen.

Symptoms continued and two weeks later Paul presented at the emergency department where he was diagnosed with complete Achilles tendon rupture.

Commentary

Dr. du Vivier was deceived by the availability bias when he was seduced by the vivid image of a ruptured tendon and assumed that if the Achilles tendon were ruptured, he would be able to palpate it. Here the availability bias did not suggest a diagnosis but suggested unrealistic reliability for a diagnostic test.

The doctor compounded the availability bias with the confirmatory bias when he maintained his assumption of the reliability of palpation despite noting the calf swelling which would have diminished the reliability of this examination.

The most effective tests for Achilles tendon rupture are the Thompson ("Calf Squeeze") Test and the Matles Test. The Thompson test has a specificity of 0.93 and a sensitivity of 0.96 (for more on sensitivity and specificity, see Chapter 20). The Matles test has a specificity of 0.85 and a sensitivity of 0.88 (Maffulli 1998). A negative result on both these tests almost guarantees an intact Achilles tendon. But du Vivier did not perform these maneuvers; he instead accepted the results of the gap palpation test, which has a sensitivity of only 0.73, and probably less if there is marked swelling.

Dr. Prasad was influenced by the availability bias in it's more conventional form when he concurred with Dr. de Vivier's diagnosis, despite the fact that three and a half weeks had progressed with no improvement. Thus, Dr. Prasad, like Dr. Ellsworth in the previous case, became a victim of "diagnosis momentum."

The availability and confirmatory biases cost the unfortunate badminton player over a month's delay in his surgical repair and possibly a suboptimal result.

Availability and Confirmatory Bias Countermeasures

Specific countermeasures to biases are necessary because, as the referenced psychological studies indicate, decision makers are frequently unaware of the biases affecting them. Biases are not simply moral lapses or character flaws to be addressed with a simple vague admonition to "Wake up and pay attention!" Instead, biases require countermeasures that are precise, simple, and reliably implemented.

Availability Bias Countermeasures

One of the most effective countermeasures to the availability bias is the formulation of a **representative list of differential diagnoses**. Generating such a diagnosis list helps ensure that the first available diagnosis is not selected and then pursued unthinkingly and unreasonably. The differential list does not need to be exhaustive; it does need to be sufficient to interrupt a spontaneous attachment to the most available diagnosis while simultaneously offering alternative diagnoses. It is at once a breaker of "bad momentum" and a generator of good alternatives.

A representative differential diagnosis list is difficult because the availability bias gives excessive weight to one's past experiences and easily recalled examples.

Consequently, in general practice, where serious conditions are less frequent, the availability bias is more likely to promote relatively benign diagnoses. On the other hand, in specialty practice, where serious conditions are more frequent, the availability bias is more likely to promote serious diagnoses (Barraclough 2013, p. 16). The management of availability bias by consideration of a representative differential diagnosis list requires **input to the list from both generalist and specialist physicians**.

Another useful countermeasure involves the **prioritizing of differential diagnoses**. The position of a diagnosis in the list of differentials itself creates an availability bias. Why not make that bias work in favor of better medical decision making? Murtagh recommends that the first diagnosis in the list should not be the most frequent diagnosis, but the one the physician cannot afford to miss (Murtagh 1990).

A final countermeasure to the availability bias involves directly **quoting the patient instead of paraphrasing**. The inclination to paraphrase may be strong because the physician's paraphrase usually involves clear, medically defined terms as an improvement over the patient's vague terminology. However, the physician's paraphrase also carries with it the possibility of infiltration by the availability bias.

Confirmatory Bias Countermeasures

A useful countermeasure to the confirmatory bias is the **double-blind study** (Novella 2012, p. 119). Such a study is frequently used to test the effectiveness of drugs. Here neither the patient nor the nurse administering the drug knows if the administered substance is the experimental drug or the control (either placebo or established drug). This reduces the possibility of the knowledge of the expected effects of the experimental drug from influencing the collection of data and, therefore, the conclusions of the study.

Another important countermeasure to the confirmatory bias is the use of objective, quantitative, **specific outcome measures**. In serial observations of patients, it is important to avoid vaguely concluding that there has been improvement, but rather to record that temperature is down, swelling as indicated by measured limb circumference is reduced, or that WBC count is decreased. This helps keep an expectation that the patient will improve from biasing the conclusion.

Orderly data collection is a useful tool to avoid the unintentional selection of confirmatory data and de-selection of dis-confirmatory data. It manifests itself in forms and protocols to be followed for recording histories, physical exams, and progress notes.

Forms and protocols should have an optimum amount of structure. Total lack of structure fails to protect against the confirmatory bias's tendency toward selection and de-selection. It also fails to call attention to areas that are innocently overlooked. Excessive structure is overwhelming and again conduces to falling back upon the confirmatory bias's tendency toward selection and de-selection. It also is conducive to automatic ticking of boxes without appropriate attention to the activity the boxes are meant to verify.

Multiple Bias Countermeasures

Background suppression or **background challenge** is a countermeasure to both availability and confirmatory biases. Cardiologist Dr. James Lock at Boston Children's Hospital described it to Dr. Jerome Groopman thus, "When a case first arrives, I don't want to hear anyone else's diagnosis. I look at the primary data" (Groopman 2008, p. 146). Although it is not possible in practice to completely suppress background information, at least challenging the background information provides some countermeasure to availability and confirmatory biases.

Consensus of scientific opinion is an effective countermeasure to multiple biases. The consensus is much more likely to be unbiased than individual opinion because in a group the biases average out and gaps in knowledge compensate for one another (Novella 2012, p. 184; Surowiecki 2014, p. 124). Nevertheless, this relative freedom from bias occurs only when the opinions forming the consensus are truly independent. If, however, multiple studies contributing to the consensus come from the same investigators, the same institution, or are funded by the same source, the independence and therefore the freedom from bias is compromised.

Conclusion

The availability and confirmatory biases often appear together. The availability bias was initially noted by Kahneman and Tversky in 1973 and the confirmatory bias was noted by Francis Bacon in 1620. Both biases have a wealth of experimental psychological investigations substantiating them. Both biases can influence physicians to unintentionally make poor medical decisions. Both biases can be better addressed as *patterns* of poor medical decision-making than as *individual* sloppiness. Both biases can be addressed by measures that are precise, simple, and reliably implemented.

References

Barraclough, K. (2013). *Avoiding errors in general practice*. Chichester, West Sussex: Wiley-Blackwell.

Chabris, C. F., & Simons, D. J. (2012). *The invisible gorilla: and other ways our intuitions deceive us*. New York: MJF Books.

Crowley, R. S., Legowski, E., Medvedeva, O., Reitmeyer, K., Tseytlin, E., Castine, M., . . . Mello-Thoms, C. (2012). Automated detection of heuristics and biases among pathologists in a computer-based system. *Advances in Health Sciences Education, 18*(3), 343-363. doi:10.1007/s10459-012-9374-z

Darley, J. M., & Fazio, R. H. (1980). Expectancy confirmation processes arising in the social interaction sequence. *American Psychologist, 35*(10), 867-881. doi:10.1037//0003-066x.35.10.867

Darley, J. M., & Gross, P. H. (1983). A hypothesis-confirming bias in labeling effects. *Journal of Personality and Social Psychology, 44*(1), 20-33. doi:10.1037//0022-3514.44.1.20

Goldacre, B. (2010). Bad science: quacks, hacks and big pharma -- flacks --. New York: Faber and Faber.

Groopman, J. E. (2010). *How doctors think*. Carlton North, Vic.: Scribe Publications.

Haines, D. (2013). Kevin Barraclough, Jenny du Toit, Jeremy Budd, Joseph E. Raine, Kate Williams and Jonathan Bonser, Avoiding errors in general practice. *Medico-Legal Journal, 81*(3), 145-145. doi:10.1177/0025817213498198

Honda, H., Shimizu, Y., & Rutter, M. (2005). No effect of MMR withdrawal on the incidence of autism: a total population study. *Journal of Child Psychology and Psychiatry, 46*(6), 572-579. doi:10.1111/j.1469-7610.2005.01425.x

Kader, D., Mosconi, M., Benazzo, F., & Maffulli, N. (n.d.). Achilles Tendon Rupture. *Tendon Injuries,* 187-200. doi:10.1007/1-84628-050-8_20

Kahneman, D. (2015). *Thinking, fast and slow*. New York: Farrar, Straus and Giroux.

Lichtenstein, S., Slovic, P., Fischhoff, B., Layman, M., & Combs, B. (1978). Judged frequency of lethal events. *Journal of Experimental Psychology: Human Learning and Memory, 4*(6), 551-578. doi:10.1037/0278-7393.4.6.551

Madsen, K. M., Hviid, A., Vestergaard, M., et al. (2002)

Measles, Mumps, and Rubella Vaccination and Autism. (2003). New England Journal of Medicine, 347(19). doi:10.1056/nejm200303063481016

Maffulli (1998). The clinical diagnosis of subcutaneous tear of the Achilles tendon. A prospective study in 174 patients. *Am J Sports Med.* 1998 Mar-Apr;26(2):266-70.

Murtagh J. (n.d.). Common problems: a safe diagnostic strategy. *Aust Fam Physician.* 1990 May;19(5):733-4, 737, 740-2.

Nickerson, R. S. (1998). Confirmation bias: A ubiquitous phenomenon in many guises. *Review of General Psychology, 2*(2), 175-220. doi:10.1037//1089-2680.2.2.175

Novella, S. (2012). *Your Deceptive Mind.* Lecture. The Great Courses.

Acute Sinusitis. (2017, January 05). Retrieved March 26, 2017, from http://emedicine.medscape.com/article/232670-overview

Schwarz, N., Bless, H., Strack, F., Klumpp, G., & Al, E. (1991). Ease of retrieval as information: Another look at the availability heuristic. *Journal of Personality and Social Psychology, 61*(2), 195-202. doi:10.1037//0022-3514.61.2.195

Shermer, M. (2012). *The believing brain: from ghosts and gods to politics and conspiracies--how we construct beliefs and reinforce them as truths.* New York: St. Martin's Griffin.

Shermer, Michael. The Believing Brain: From Ghosts and Gods to Politics and Conspiracies---How We Construct Beliefs and Reinforce Them as Truths (p. 363). Henry Holt and Co.. Kindle Edition.

Simel, D. L., Keitz, S. A., & Rennie, D. (2009). *The Rational clinical examination: evidence-based clinical diagnosis.* New York: McGraw-Hill Medical/JAMA & Archives Journals.

Surowiecki, J. (2014). *The wisdom of crowds why the many are smarter than the few.* London: Abacus.

Tversky, A., & Kahneman, D. (1973). Availability: A heuristic for judging frequency and probability. *Cognitive Psychology, 5*(2), 207-232. doi:10.1016/0010-0285(73)90033-9

Further Reading

Barraclough, K. (2013). *Avoiding errors in general practice*. Chichester, West Sussex: Wiley-Blackwell.

Chabris, C. F., & Simons, D. J. (2012). *The invisible gorilla: and other ways our intuitions deceive us*. New York: MJF Books.

Goldacre, B. (2010). Bad science: quacks, hacks and big pharma -- flacks --. New York: Faber and Faber.

Groopman, J. E. (2010). *How doctors think*. Carlton North, Vic.: Scribe Publications.
Kahneman, D. (2015). *Thinking, fast and slow*. New York: Farrar, Straus and Giroux.

Novella, S. (2012). Your deceptive mind: a scientific guide to critical thinking skills. Chantilly, VA: Teaching Company.

Shermer, Michael. The Believing Brain: From Ghosts and Gods to Politics and Conspiracies---How We Construct Beliefs and Reinforce Them as Truths (p. 363). Henry Holt and Co.. Kindle Edition.

Simel, D. L., Keitz, S. A., & Rennie, D. (2009). *The Rational clinical examination: evidence-based clinical diagnosis*. New York: McGraw-Hill Medical/JAMA & Archives Journals.

Chapter 5: Blind Spot and Overconfidence Biases

Although all biases tend to operate below the threshold of attention, the **bias-blind-spot bias** and the **overconfidence bias** are particularly insidious. Other biases compromise judgment and decision-making; but these two biases compromise the ability to recognize that judgment and decision-making are compromised. The bias-blind-spot bias does this by hiding the primary bias. The overconfidence bias does this by intensifying the primary bias to the point that alternatives seem non-existent. Therefore, the bias-blind-spot bias and overconfidence bias are second-order or meta-biases.

Blind-Spot Bias

The **bias-blind-spot bias** is an influence hiding a primary bias from the person affected by the primary bias. It is the tendency to see bias in other people but not in oneself. Like other biases, it operates below the level of attention.

Common Example – Blind-Spot Bias

Of all drivers surveyed, 83% regarded use of cell phones while driving as a serious or very serious traffic safety problem. Nevertheless, of these, 29-46% reported having used their cell phone while driving at least occasionally in the preceding 30 days (Traffic Safety Culture Index 2008). Add to this the study indicating that 93% of American drivers rated themselves as better than median (Svenson 1981), and it suggests that **drivers regard themselves at least partially immune to the inattention bias** that they find so common in others.

Pronin Experiments – Blind-Spot Bias

Pronin and colleagues performed several experiments in 2002.

First, they asked 23 Stanford students involved in an upper-level psychology seminar to study a booklet describing eight specific cognitive biases. They then asked them to rate on a 9-point scale their own susceptibility to these biases versus the susceptibility of the "average American." The students reported themselves less susceptible than the "Average American."

Second, the researchers repeated the experiment the following year with 30 students from the same-level class. This time they asked the students to compare their own bias-susceptibility with that of their classmates. Although the difference was less, the students still rated themselves less bias-susceptible than their peers.

Third, the Pronin researchers performed a similar experiment with 76 persons of various ages and ethnic backgrounds awaiting flights at San Francisco International Airport (SFO). They asked the subjects to compare their own bias-susceptibility versus the bias-susceptibility of the other SFO travelers. Again, the subjects rated themselves less bias-susceptible than their fellow travelers.

Fourth, the same researchers asked 91 Stanford students to rate themselves on a 9-point scale "relative to other Stanford students" on objectivity and five other personality dimensions. The experimenters then presented the subjects with a description of the "better-than-average" bias (overconfidence bias), which included the statement "70-80% of individuals consistently rate themselves better-than-average."

The subjects were then told that for purposes of the study, it would be useful to know the accuracy of the self-assessments they had just made. Accordingly, the subjects were asked to indicate how they thought they would be rated by the "most accurate, valid, and objective resources available": a) lower on positive characteristics and higher on negative ones, b) higher on positive and lower on negative, or c) no differently than they had rated themselves.

As results, 24% indicated that they had claimed better status than warranted, 63% reported that their self-evaluation was accurate and objective, and 13% indicated that their self-evaluation had been *too modest*.

Even after exposure to putative information that 70-80% of subjects consistently over-rate themselves, 76% regarded their self-evaluation as accurate and valid or as too modest (Pronin 2002).

Medical Examples and Steinman Experiment – Blind-Spot Bias

The **bias-blind-spot bias occurs significantly among patients afflicted with alcoholism**. The alcoholic patient often contends that he is a heavy drinker but not an alcoholic. He claims that alcoholics erroneously think that they can stop drinking when, in fact, they cannot. He contends, that he, on the other hand, *could stop drinking any time he wished*, but that he just does not so desire (Treating Addiction 2017). In effect, the alcoholic patient contends that others are subject to the **illusion of control bias** but that he is not.

Lack of insight attributable to the bias-blind-spot bias applies to physicians as well as patients.

Steinman and colleagues did a study involving 105 resident physicians concerning the **acceptance by physicians of gifts** such as pens and lunches from pharmaceutical company representatives. While 61% of the physicians stated that the acceptance of such gifts did not influence their own prescribing habits, only 16% stated that other physicians were so immune (Steinman 2001). They were more cognizant of the presence of the **self-serving bias** in other physicians but less cognizant of its presence in themselves.

Countermeasures to the Blind-Spot Bias

The bias-blind-spot bias is particularly insidious as *it is difficult to devise countermeasures to a bias that is almost invisible*. Nevertheless, some measures exist. Since these are also countermeasures to the overconfidence bias, their discussion will follow the examination of the overconfidence bias.

Overconfidence Bias

Overconfidence bias is a tendency to overestimate one's abilities especially regarding difficult tasks.

The overconfidence bias seems to be a **consequence of not knowing the unknown unknowns**, their existence, their content, and their application to the problem. When insight into the lack of knowledge is missing, overconfidence in existing knowledge goes unchastened.

In consequence, those who are less informed are often more confident. In this regard, Kahneman explains, "the consistency of information matters a great deal for assent, and **knowing little makes it easier to achieve consistency**" (Kahneman 2015, p. 87).

Finally, the **overconfidence bias can exert its influence several times sequentially** in the consideration of a single problem. Overconfidence can intervene in the validity of the information, again in the understanding of the information, again in the accuracy of recall of the information, and once more in the appropriate application of the information.

Common Examples – Overconfidence Bias

Chess players in tournament play are assigned a point rating by the US Chess Federation. Chess masters are those with a rating of 2200 points or higher. If a player beats or ties a higher-rated player in a tournament, his point rating increases and his opponent's point rating decreases.

Chabris surveyed 103 players in tournaments in Philadelphia, PA and Parsippany, NJ. He found that weaker players thought that they were underrated by an average of 150 points while stronger players thought that they were underrated by an average of 50 points (Chabris 2012, p.88).

Svenson studied **American drivers** and found that 93% rated themselves as better than the median (Svenson 1981).

Common Example and Kruger-Dunning Experiments – Overconfidence Bias

Kruger and Dunning begin their paper with the story of MacArthur Wheeler who in 1995 robbed two Pittsburgh banks in broad daylight with no attempted disguise. He was arrested that night an hour after pictures of him on surveillance camera were telecast on the 11PM news.

When arrested, Wheeler was incredulous and mumbled, "But I wore the juice." He was certain that rubbing his face with lemon juice made him invisible to the closed circuit TV cameras!

Kruger and Dunning tested subjects in four experiments: one in humor, one in grammar, and two in logic. They had the subjects estimate their performance on these tasks. While the subjects scored in only the 12th percentile, they estimated their own performance as being in the 62nd percentile (Kruger 1999).

Medical Examples of the Overconfidence Bias

Friedman and his group selected medical cases to examine the diagnostic accuracy of attending physicians, residents, and medical students. They then compared this accuracy with the subjects' confidence in the diagnoses they made.

Their findings were that the medical students were the least accurate and the least confident. The attending physicians were the most accurate and the most confident. However, the residents were less accurate in their diagnoses than the attending physicians but were more confident (Friedman 2005).

Potchen compared diagnostic accuracy against confidence in 95 board-certified radiologists. The aggregate accuracy of the top 20 radiologists was 95% versus

75% for the bottom 20. Nevertheless, the worst performers had a higher confidence level than the best performers (Potchen 2006).

Countermeasures to the Overconfidence Bias

The first countermeasure depends on the fact that the *less competent* are the *more confident*. It therefore recommends **improving competence** (Chabris 2012, p. 107). Of course, this is not an easy fix; but it is a double win: First, it increases accuracy, and second, it increases awareness of residual inaccuracy.

The second countermeasure should be easier to implement and maintain. This countermeasure addresses the fact that the lesser trained, lesser experienced, worse performing personnel have a higher confidence level. These are individual more likely in subordinate positions.

The measure simply requires that managers of subordinates prepare a **comprehensive, detailed, unambiguous, written list of responsibilities** that can be assigned to the subordinates. The list should be **objectively calibrated**, documented, **signed by all participants**, and subject to frequent review and feedback on effectiveness. This measure can help address overconfidence among those who are less trained and less experienced.

On the other hand, the overconfidence bias can affect supervisors as well as subordinates. In this case, the supervisors may contend, "I am confident in my people's capabilities and they know their comfort zone. Besides, they know that I am available whenever they think that they are in over their heads." In this case, the written, objectively calibrated, periodically reviewed list of responsibilities and competencies can chasten the overconfidence of supervisors as well as subordinates.

Countermeasures to the Blind-Spot and Overconfidence Biases

The first countermeasure to the blind spot and overconfidence biases is **adequate reference to the population base-rate**. If the resident physicians in Steinman's study had been randomly selected and making estimates of themselves according to the base-rate of their own population, they would have judged themselves more closely resembling the 61% than the 16%. If the underperforming radiologists in the Potchen study had estimated their confidence from the base-rate of radiologist accuracy, their assessments would have been more precise than when taken from their introspection.

A second countermeasure to the blind spot and overconfidence biases is also a countermeasure to the confirmatory bias. This countermeasure, proposed by

Daniel Kahneman, consists of **projecting one year into the future after the decision was made and imagining the decision was a disaster**. Kahneman's technique encourages writing a brief history of the disaster. Doing so, when done privately, functions as a countermeasure to the blind spot bias, overconfidence bias, and confirmatory bias. When done publically, as part of pre-established procedure, it serves to avoid the appearance of disloyalty and legitimizes doubts (Kahneman 2015, pp. 264-266).

Conclusion

The bias-blind-spot bias and the overconfidence bias are particularly insidious because they compromise the ability to recognize that judgment and decision-making are compromised. However, the countermeasures to these biases should help alleviate the problems of a little knowledge being a dangerous thing and of not knowing what one does not know!

References

2008 Traffic Safety Culture Index. (n.d.). PsycEXTRA Dataset. doi:10.1037/e557532012-001

Chabris, C. F., & Simons, D. J. (2012). *The invisible gorilla: and other ways our intuitions deceive us*. New York: MJF Books.

Cognitive bias. (2017, April 09). Retrieved April 11, 2017, from https://en.wikipedia.org/wiki/Cognitive_bias

Davis, D. A., Mazmanian, P. E., Fordis, M., Harrison, R. V., Thorpe, K. E., & Perrier, L. (2006). Accuracy of Physician Self-assessment Compared With Observed Measures of Competence. *Jama, 296*(9), 1094. doi:10.1001/jama.296.9.1094

Friedman, C. P., Gatti, G. G., Franz, T. M., Murphy, G. C., Wolf, F. M., Heckerling, P. S., . . . Elstein, A. S. (2005). Do physicians know when their diagnoses are correct? *Journal of General Internal Medicine, 20*(4), 334-339. doi:10.1111/j.1525-1497.2005.30145.x

Hall, K. H. (2002). Reviewing intuitive decision-making and uncertainty: the implications for medical education. *Medical Education, 36*(3), 216-224. doi:10.1046/j.1365-2923.2002.01140.x

List of cognitive biases. (2017, March 24). Retrieved April 02, 2017, from https://en.wikipedia.org/wiki/List_of_cognitive_biases

Kahneman, D. (2015). *Thinking, fast and slow*. New York: Farrar, Straus and Giroux.

Kahneman, D., & Tversky, A. (1972). Subjective probability: A judgment of representativeness. *Cognitive Psychology, 3*(3), 430-454. doi:10.1016/0010-0285(72)90016-3

Kruger, J., & Dunning, D. (1999). Unskilled and unaware of it: How difficulties in recognizing one's own incompetence lead to inflated self-assessments. *Journal of Personality and Social Psychology, 77*(6), 1121-1134. doi:10.1037//0022-3514.77.6.1121

Mitchell, D. J., Russo, J. E., & Pennington, N. (1989). Back to the future: Temporal perspective in the explanation of events. Journal of Behavioral Decision Making,2(1), 25-38. doi:10.1002/bdm.3960020103

Moore, D. A., & Healy, P. J. (2008). The trouble with overconfidence. *Psychological Review, 115*(2), 502-517. doi:10.1037/0033-295x.115.2.502

Potchen, E. J. (2006). Measuring Observer Performance in Chest Radiology: Some Experiences. Journal of the American College of Radiology,3(6), 423-432. doi:10.1016/j.jacr.2006.02.020

Pronin, E. (2007). Perception and misperception of bias in human judgment. Trends in Cognitive Sciences,11(1), 37-43. doi:10.1016/j.tics.2006.11.001

Pronin, E., Lin, D. Y., & *Ross*, L. (2002). The Bias Blind Spot: Perceptions of Bias in Self Versus Others. *Personality and Social Psychology Bulletin, 28*(3), 369-381. doi:10.1177/0146167202286008

Redelmeier, D. A. (2005). The Cognitive Psychology of Missed Diagnoses. *Annals of Internal Medicine, 142*(2), 115. doi:10.7326/0003-4819-142-2-200501180-00010

Steinman, M. A., Shlipak, M. G., & Mcphee, S. J. (2001). Of principles and pens: attitudes and practices of medicine housestaff toward pharmaceutical industry promotions. *The American Journal of Medicine, 110*(7), 551-557. doi:10.1016/s0002-9343(01)00660-x

Svenson, O. (1981). Are we all less risky and more skillful than our fellow drivers? Acta Psychologica,47(2), 143-148. doi:10.1016/0001-6918(81)90005-6

Treating addiction. Transforming lives. (n.d.). Retrieved April 11, 2017, from http://www.hazeldenbettyford.org/

Tversky, A., & Kahneman, D. (1973). Availability: A heuristic for judging frequency and probability. *Cognitive Psychology, 5*(2), 207-232. doi:10.1016/0010-0285(73)90033-9

Further Reading

Chabris, C. F., & Simons, D. J. (2012). *The invisible gorilla: and other ways our intuitions deceive us*. New York: MJF Books.

Kahneman, D. (2015). *Thinking, fast and slow*. New York: Farrar, Straus and Giroux.

Kruger, J., & Dunning, D. (1999). Unskilled and unaware of it: How difficulties in recognizing one's own incompetence lead to inflated self-assessments. *Journal of Personality and Social Psychology, 77*(6), 1121-1134. doi:10.1037//0022-3514.77.6.1121

Chapter 6: Action Bias

Action Bias

Action bias, or **commission bias**, is a tendency toward action rather than inaction when the outcome is likely to be the same regardless of the decision. It reflects the urge to "do something" (Croskerry 2002). Worse, it may reflect the tendency to "do something NOW!"

The action bias is evident in medicine in the following (Croskerry 2002) (Foy 2013):
- The use of unnecessary medications
- The ordering of unnecessary studies
- The ordering of more aggressive studies than warranted
- The rapid adoption of interventions without sufficient evidence of effectiveness
- The persistence of interventions long after their benefit has been disproven.

Since actions undertaken under the influence of action bias involve a positive intervention, they may be less reversible than errors of omission (Croskerry 2002).

Bar-Eli Study – Action Bias

Michael Bar-Eli and colleagues studied action bias in **soccer goalkeepers** during penalty kicks. They observed whether the goalkeeper jumped left, right, or remained in the center (Bar-Eli 2007).

The investigators point out that at the position from which the penalty kick is made, the ball is only 11 meters from the goal and that this gives the goalkeeper only 0.2-0.3 seconds to act (Chiappori 2002) (Palacios-Huerta 2003). They suspected that this was insufficient time for the goalkeeper to observe kick direction and react, but, rather, that the goalkeeper must decide an action beforehand. They supported this with the observation that in the 286 cases they studied, the direction of the kick and the jump matched in 43% of kicks rather than in 100% (Bar-Eli 2007).

The Bar-Eli group then noted that the percentage of kicks to the left, right, or center were 32.2%, 39.2%, and 28.7% respectively. Further, the percentages of successful stops made by the goalie on jumping left, right, or remaining center were 14.2%, 12.6% and 33.3% respectively. Nevertheless, the percentages of times the goalie jumped left, right, or remained center were 49.3%, 44.4%, and 6.3% respectively.

In summary, kickers made 28.7% of their kicks toward the center. Goalies successfully stopped 33.3% of these, more than twice as many as they stopped when jumping either left or right. Yet, goalies remained at the center only 6.3% of the time. The Bar-Eli investigators proposed that these data are explained by goalies being influenced by the action bias (Bar-Eli 2007).

Common Example – Action Bias

Patrick Labbe is a Certified Financial Analyst who observes the commission bias in financial clients. He writes that many investors follow daily price changes and political developments so that they can quickly trade one investment for another, chasing last year's winners.

He advises that investing is not all about active trading but, rather, about time in the market with a proven investment strategy (Labbe 2017).

Medical Examples – Action Bias

Medical examples of action bias are seen in the use of antibiotics for viral illness, and the use of drugs to treat medication side effects instead of prescribing more selectively.

Another example of action bias appears in the persistent widespread use of **pulmonary artery catheterization** long after evidence mounted that failed to support benefit from such generalized use of this technology (ESCAPE Trial Investigators 2005), (Harvey 2005), (Sandham 2003), (Wheeler 2006).

A final example comes to mind when the author, as a patient received a prescription knowingly reordering the same MRI that had, just a few weeks previously, returned normal, with no technical difficulties, and with no change in symptoms.

Explanations for Action Bias

Kahneman-Tversky Study – Fear of Regret as Explanation for Action Bias

A Kahneman-Tversky study may provide some explanation of the action bias.

In their study, Kahneman and Tversky presented 138 subjects with the following scenario:

Mr. Paul owns shares in company A. During the past year, he considered switching to stock in company B, but decided against it. He now finds that he would have been better off by $1200 if he had switched the stock to company B.

Mr. George owned shares in company B. During the past year, he switched to stock in company A. He now finds that he would have been better off by $1200 if he had kept his stock in company B.

When the researchers asked the subjects, who they thought felt greater regret, 92% of subjects said Mr. George, while 8% of the subjects said Mr. Paul. The researchers concluded that **outcomes following exceptional actions might elicit stronger affective reactions than outcomes of routine actions** (Kahneman 1982).

Applying this hypothesis to the soccer goalies, it may be that the routine action is to jump left or right while the exceptional action is to remain at the center. If so, greater regret may be felt on remaining centered and failing to stop the shot than on jumping left or right and failing to stop the shot. Avoiding this greater regret, the goalies tend to jump left or right.

Defensive Medicine as Explanation for Action Bias

An often-cited explanation for excessive testing, excessive prescribing, and excessive intervention is defensive medicine prompted by the threat of litigation.

Studdert Survey

During a **medical professional liability insurance crisis in Pennsylvania** during the early 2000s, a crisis in which physicians' insurance premiums increased sharply, Studdert and colleagues made a study of defensive medicine.

Their study involved a mail survey of 1268 physicians in six specialties with the most costly insurance premiums. Of these, 824 physicians completed and returned the survey, for which they received an honorarium of $75.

In this self-reporting, the physicians responded by answering 1) never, 2) rarely, 3) sometimes, or 4) often, to questions including
- Do you order more tests than medically indicated?
- Do you prescribe more medications than medically indicated?
- Do you refer to specialists in unnecessary circumstances?
- Do you suggest invasive procedures against professional judgment?

- Do you avoid doing certain procedures?
- Do you avoid treating high-risk patients?

In all, 93% of the respondents indicated that they sometimes or often engaged in one of the above six types of defensive medicine. Specifically, 52% of respondents indicated that they often ordered unnecessary consultations or referrals. Additionally, 63% of emergency physicians, 41% of general surgeons, 55% of orthopedic surgeons, and 58% of neurosurgeons reported ordering unnecessary CTs, MRIs, or x-rays.

Finally, 42% reported that liability concerns had caused them to eliminate some types of procedures they had been offering and that they were now avoiding some patients with complex medical problems or those perceived to be litigious. An additional 7% reported that they were likely to take these actions in the next two years (Studdert 2005).

However, below are the **problems with surveys in general and with the Studdert survey in particular**:
- Of those contacted, 35% did not respond. Nonresponders are rarely random; they may not respond for reasons that impact the conclusions of the study.
- Self-reporters may not actually report their actions but rather report the way they wish they had acted or the way they think it would have been appropriate to act.
- The study was not blinded and the subjects were clearly vulnerable to outcome bias. They knew that their responses could be used as evidence that litigation was causing costly, unnecessary procedures and was encouraging physicians to reduce types of care offered.
- The subjects also knew that this survey was being conducted in the midst of a professional liability insurance crisis. They knew that the survey results could be used to support legislation to reduce the volume of litigation and thereby lower the respondents' runaway insurance premiums.

Klingman Study

As early as the mid 1990s, Klingman and colleagues had concerns about using self-reporting physician surveys to study the extent of defensive medicine. Instead, they **offered their subjects a set of clinical scenarios and tabulated their choices of action** (Klingman 1996).

The Klingman investigators determined that defensive medicine existed to a much lesser extent than expected. They found that in all the scenarios, the majority of physicians chose aggressive patient management even though conservative management was considered medically acceptable. Perceived medical indications, rather than liability concerns, motivated their clinical choices. Only about 8% of interventions seemed to be undertaken predominantly as defensive medicine measures.

As an example, the Klingman investigators pointed out that 60% of cardiologists indicated they would order either an exercise EKG or stress thallium study on a healthy, active 42 year-old man who presented to the ER with non-cardiac chest pain (i.e., pain on rotation of the left shoulder). The subjects indicated they would do this even if the patient had no risk factors for coronary artery disease (CAD), a normal EKG, and negative cardiac enzymes (Foy 2013).

It seems that factors additional to defensive medicine are necessary to explain action bias.

Self-interest Bias

Self-interest bias certainly seems to contribute to action bias. The self-interests especially appealed to are financial and self-esteem.

Financial Self-interest

The **traditional model for health care reimbursement financially rewards procedures and thus inspires increasing medical interventions**. This continues until the limits of the health care budget are approached. Then, to contain the health care budget, reimbursements for individual interventions begin to be reduced. However, the mentality of procedures has already been established, and the equipment and facilities for performing them have already been heavily invested in. Consequently, so long as reimbursements do not fall too much too quickly, the tendency is to make up for declining individual reimbursements by performing ever more procedures.

Self-esteem

Physicians' self-esteem may well be enhanced by the action bias. A **feeling of accomplishment and self-value accompanies the successful completion of an intervention**. This feeling is an instantaneous reward and may certainly fuel the action bias.

Moral Hazard

Foy describes moral hazard as a contributing factor to action bias (Foy 2013).

He cites a study showing that **a fully insured population spends about 40% to 50% more than a population with a large deductible** and that their status is not measurably improved by the additional services (Manning 1987).

Certainly, it is never a good reason to get a study or intervention just because it is available with no co-pay or at a markedly reduced co-pay.

Patient Pressure

Patients are also influenced by the action bias. Consequently, they **may pressure physicians to prescribe the latest drug** advertised on television, to order tests and radiographic studies, or to make specialist referrals. The physicians often comply.

In one study 36% of physicians told researchers that they would yield to a patient who asked for a clinically unwarranted magnetic resonance imaging exam (Foy 2013).

In a survey of 51,946 adults conducted between 2000 and 2007, respondents in the highest quartile of patient satisfaction had higher odds of inpatient admission, greater total expenditures, and greater prescription drug expenditures (Fenton 2012).

Consequences of the Action Bias

The three main **negative consequences of action bias are poor use of resources, patient exposure to iatrogenic injury, and corruption of medical data**.

It comes as no surprise that health care resources are finite. Every dollar that is spent ill advisedly on one diagnostic study, intervention, or medication is a dollar that is unavailable to other patients for truly needed health care.

Further, diagnostic studies and interventions are not without risk, and medications are not without side effects. Unnecessary activities might satisfy the action bias of the doctor but may be detrimental to the patient.

Finally, overuse of treatments can corrupt data. Drugs and interventions can do well in early studies on well-defined patients. However, as they become more popular, they may tend to be used in marginal patients with less firm diagnoses. This can lead to their seeming to become less efficacious.

Countermeasures to the Action Bias

Croskerry suggests that, before acting, **physicians ask themselves a few questions**:
- Is the action justified?
- What are the consequences of the action?
- Is there an associated danger?
- Are there other options?
- Is the action revocable?
- How much of the action can be reversed? (Croskerry 2002)

We suggest, as additional countermeasures to the action bias, **some "Do not"s and some "Do"s**:
- Do not assume that doing ANYTHING is better than doing nothing.
- Do not succumb to the technology bias or to the novelty bias.
- Do not implement an action because it is available or available at a discount.
- Identify what you expect from a study, intervention, or medication before proceeding.
- Plan ahead what you will do if the test is positive or negative, if the drug works or not.
- Reconsider a test or intervention if it will not make a difference in the patient's treatment.
- Always consider the complications of an intervention, the side effects of a drug, or limitations of a diagnostic test.
- Be aware that excessive testing may be a litigation exposure as well as a litigation defense. Pursuing false positives may lead to complications. Not pursuing them may raise the suspicion of negligence.
- Be aware of your own self-interest motivations and needs: money, validation, etc.
- Consider if actions can be safely deferred until later; they may prove to be unnecessary.
- Develop an "exit strategy" if a decision goes wrong.

Conclusion

The **action bias** is often tied to the availability bias, the overconfidence bias, and the confirmatory bias. It potentiates these biases by moving them into action, and doing so with a velocity that precludes critical reflection. It satisfies some visceral impulses in the physician but does not serve the best interests of the patient. Fortunately, the action bias is one against which many effective countermeasures can be mobilized. These can sometimes be embodied in the aphorism "If it isn't broken, don't fix it!"

References

Bar-Eli, M. (2007, January 25). Action bias among elite soccer goalkeepers: The case of penalty kicks. Retrieved November 22, 2017, from https://www.sciencedirect.com/science/article/pii/S0167487006001048

Chiappori, P., Levitt, S., & Groseclose, T. (2002). Testing Mixed-Strategy Equilibria When Players Are Heterogeneous: The Case of Penalty Kicks in Soccer. *American Economic Review,92*(4), 1138-1151. doi:10.1257/00028280260344678

Croskerry, P. (2002). Achieving Quality in Clinical Decision Making: Cognitive Strategies and Detection of Bias. *Academic Emergency Medicine, 9*(11), 1184-1204. doi:10.1197/aemj.9.11.1184

ESCAPE Trial Investigators. (2005). Evaluation Study of Congestive Heart Failure and Pulmonary Artery Catheterization Effectiveness. *Jama,294*(13), 1625. doi:10.1001/jama.294.13.1625

Fenton, J. J. (2012). The Cost of Satisfaction. *Archives of Internal Medicine,172*(5), 405-411. doi:10.1001/archinternmed.2011.1662

Foy, A. (spring 2013). Don't Just Do Something, Stand There! Intervention Bias in Medical Decision Making. *Journal of American Physicians and Surgeons, 18*(1), 17-21. Retrieved November 26, 2017.

Harvey, S., Harrison, D. A., Singer, M., Ashcroft, J., Jones, C. M., Elbourne, D., . . . Rowan, K. (2005). Assessment of the clinical effectiveness of pulmonary artery catheters in management of patients in intensive care (PAC-Man): a randomised controlled trial. *The Lancet,366*(9484), 472-477. doi:10.1016/s0140-6736(05)67061-4

Kahneman, D., & Tversky, A. (1982). The simulation heuristic. *Judgment under uncertainty,*201-208. doi:10.1017/cbo9780511809477.015

Kahneman, D., & Miller, D. T. (1986). Norm Theory: Comparing Reality to Its Alternatives. *Psychological Review,93*(2), 136-153. doi:10.1017/cbo9780511808098.022

Kahneman, D. (2015). *Thinking, fast and slow*. New York: Farrar, Straus and Giroux.

Klingman, D., Localio, A. R., Sugarman, J., Wagner, J. L., Polishuk, P. T., Wolfe, L., & Corrigan, J. A. (1996). Measuring Defensive Medicine Using Clinical Scenario Surveys. *Journal of Health Politics, Policy and Law,21*(2), 185-220. doi:10.1215/03616878-21-2-185

Labbe, P. (n.d.). Our Bias Toward Action INVESTING BEHAVIORAL FINANCE. Retrieved November 22, 2017, from https://www.jvbruni.com/articles/our-bias-toward-action

Manning, Newhouse, & Duan. (1987). Health insurance and the demand for medical care: evidence from a randomized experiment. *Am Economic ,77*, 251-277.

Palacios-Huerta, I. (2003). Professionals Play Minimax. *Review of Economic Studies,70*(2), 395-415. doi:10.1111/1467-937x.00249

Sandham, Hull, & Brant. (2003). Pulmonary-Artery Catheters in High-Risk Surgical Patients. *New England Journal of Medicine,348*(20), 2035-2037. doi:10.1056/nejm200305153482019

Studdert, D. M. (2005). Defensive Medicine Among High-Risk Specialist Physicians in a Volatile Malpractice Environment. *Jama,293*(21), 2609. doi:10.1001/jama.293.21.2609

Wheeler, Bernard, & Thompson. (2006). Pulmonary-Artery versus Central Venous Catheter to Guide Treatment of Acute Lung Injury. *New England Journal of Medicine,354*(21), 2213-2224. doi:10.1056/nejmoa061895

Further Reading

Croskerry, P. (2002). Achieving Quality in Clinical Decision Making: Cognitive Strategies and Detection of Bias. *Academic Emergency Medicine, 9*(11), 1184-1204. doi:10.1197/aemj.9.11.1184

Kahneman, D. (2015). *Thinking, fast and slow*. New York: Farrar, Straus and Giroux.

Chapter 7: Planning Fallacy

Planning Fallacy

Planning fallacy, or **planning bias,** was first identified by Daniel Kahneman and Amos Tversky in a technical report for the US Defense Advanced Research Projects Agency (Kahneman 1977). In that report, the authors characterized planning bias as the tendency to underestimate the time required for completion of a project, even when the planners have considerable experience of past failures, and even when underestimation of duration or cost is penalized.

In a subsequent paper (Lovallo 2003), Lovallo and Kahneman expanded that definition, characterizing it as an *optimistic tendency to predict success while overlooking the potential for mistakes and miscalculations*.

Origins of Planning Fallacy

The planning fallacy finds some of its origins in the overconfidence bias, the anchoring bias, confirmatory bias, and organizational pressure.

Overconfidence bias has been discussed previously; and, it is obvious how overconfidence would lead to optimism in the ability to realize a plan.

Anchoring bias, also previously discussed, makes its presence felt when the initial plan poses such a substantial anchor that conscious allowances and adjustments from it are insufficient to model the real situation.

Confirmatory bias is especially dangerous in planning. It focuses on the positive information supporting how things will go right with the plan. It minimizes negative information about the known unknowns that can disrupt the plan.

Isolation of probabilities is another contributor to the planning fallacy. The probability of a single rare event *not occurring* is very high. But the probability of an entire group of rare events *not occurring* is the *product* of all the probabilities. So all the individual probabilities, each less than 1.0, multiply when the events become part of a complicated plan. The probability of a particular adverse event *not occurring* may be high, but the probability of no adverse event occurring may be low.

Unknown unknowns are yet one more contributor to the planning fallacy. First, one can consider entropy and statistical mechanics to realize that there are many, many more possible disorganized states than there are possible organized states. That is, there are multitudinous ways for a plan to fail and only a few ways for a plan to succeed. Second, one can consider chaos theory to realize that even small differences in early conditions can result in vast differences in later conditions, making later conditions incredibly difficult to anticipate.

Common Example – Planning Fallacy

Kahneman cites a personal example of the planning fallacy.

He was leading a team to **design a curriculum to teach decision making in Israeli high schools**. The team estimated that the project would require two years. Kahneman then asked his associate Seymour Fox for data on other teams working on similar projects. Fox reported that 40% of the teams never finished the project and that the ones that did finish took between seven and ten years. The team disregarded this data and clung to their original estimate of two years.

The result was that the project required eight years. By the time it was completed, the ministry of Education lost interest in the project, and the completed project was never implemented (Kahneman 2015, pp 245-247).

Medical Examples – Planning Fallacy

Planning Fallacy – Travis Study

The planning fallacy seems to play out every day in the operating room, as evidenced by the Travis study.

Travis and her group conducted a prospective observation of orthopedic surgeons, plastic surgeons, general surgeons, and anesthesiologists. They compared the time estimates given by the physicians immediately before their respective procedures began with the time the procedures actually took. The investigators found that orthopedic surgeons *overpredicted* their procedure time by an average of 1.0%. However, plastic **surgeons *underpredicted* their procedure time** by 4.3%, general surgeons by 28.7%, and anesthesiologists by 62.6%.

Planning Fallacy – Surgical Case

A patient **lived out of town but was undergoing a trial for an implanted intrathecal catheter** with morphine pump for control of intractable pain. The catheter was inserted in the operating room under sterile conditions and the pump, with antibacterial filter at the catheter – pump tubing connection was connected. The physician preferred that the patient stay in town for the three days of the trial. The patient desired to return home and be checked by his local visiting nurses.

The physician only needed the visiting nurses to visit daily for the three day trial; record the patient's pain level; daily observe, but not touch, the catheter, connections, or dressing; record if the dressing was dry but phone the physician if it was wet. The physician checked with the visiting nurses, who assured him they could do this.

On the third day, already the day scheduled for removal, the patient presented at the emergency department with a severe headache. The physician aspirated the intrathecal catheter and noted cloudy spinal fluid. The patient had bacterial meningitis. Fortunately, the patient recovered.

On questioning the patient, the physician later learned that one of the visiting nurses, contrary to instructions, had disconnected and reconnected the catheter, under nonsterile conditions, below the level of the antibacterial filter.

What could have gone wrong with such a simple plan? The visiting nurse supervisors could have overrated the capabilities of their staff. Because of scheduling problems, the contacted supervisors could have communicated only through intermediaries with the nurses actually attending the patient. The attending nurse could have misunderstood instructions. Attending nurses could have switched assignments to reduce redundant travel. The attending nurse could have been replaced by an uninstructed substitute when she was sick, had a family emergency, or was involved in an auto accident. The unknown unknowns are numerous.

Countermeasures – Planning Fallacy

Kahneman and Tversky, in addition to identifying the planning fallacy, have also advanced a countermeasure called *reference class forecasting* (Kahneman 1977) (Kahneman 2015). The idea here is that the unknown unknowns cannot be measured or even identified but perhaps their effects can be assessed.

The **first step is to identify an appropriate similar reference class and to develop from this the statistics of the reference class to make a baseline prediction**.

Sometimes this is easier than others. If the plan is to write a book, one can easily select a reference class of books on the same topic, develop from this class the means and standard deviations for numerous parameters, and then use these to get a more accurate projection of those parameters, such as likelihood of completion, number of copies sold, etc.

Sometimes this is more difficult. Let us return to our example of the visiting nurses attending the patient having an intrathecal morphine trial. One might need to develop information on visiting nurse services tasked with simple but unfamiliar projects. One might then need to develop data on initial task accomplishment with no problems, minimal problems, significant problems, and life-threatening problems. Calculating means and standard deviations, one might be able to use this to estimate probabilities of success with the envisioned new task.

The **second step is to use specific information about the particular case to adjust the baseline prediction**, bearing in mind that the baseline prediction is to be adjusted, not abrogated.

Conclusion

The planning fallacy is stealthy. While it springs from other biases, it adds the element of the unknown unknowns. However, it is somewhat tractable if one avoids being preoccupied with details of the plan and instead focuses on the statistical properties of a representative class to which the plan belongs.

References

Kahneman, D., & Tversky, A. (June 1977). Intuitive prediction: Biases and corrective procedures. *Report to Defense Advanced Research Projects Agency*. doi:10.1017/cbo9780511809477.031

Lovallo, D., & Kahneman, D. (July 2003). Delusions of Success: How Optimism Undermines Executives' Decisions. *Harvard Business Review*.

Kahneman, D. (2015). *Thinking, fast and slow*. New York: Farrar, Straus and Giroux.

Travis, E., Woodhouse, S., Tan, R., Patel, S., Donovan, J., & Brogan, K. (2014). Operating theatre time, where does it all go? A prospective observational study. *Bmj,349*(Dec15 6). doi:10.1136/bmj.g7182

Further Reading

Kahneman, D. (2015). *Thinking, fast and slow*. New York: Farrar, Straus and Giroux.

Chapter 8: Conformity Bias

Conformity Bias

Conformity bias is a tendency to exhibit behavior similar to that of others when the specific behavior is contrary to what is exhibited without such influence. A few examples will serve to explicate this.

Common Examples of the Conformity Bias

Two instances of the conformity bias were featured on the television program *Candid Camera*. The program debuted on American television in 1948 and reprised in several iterations thereafter. The program featured pranks in which unusual social situations were constructed in an effort to determine if the subject of the prank would behave irrationally, to the amusement of the television audience.

The first prank involved an elevator. A few actors stood in the elevator car with their backs to the door. As the elevator stopped at the next floor, in a surprising number of instances, the victim of the prank would enter the car and stand with his back to the door in conformity with the other occupants.

In a second prank, a group of actors on the sidewalk of a busy street stood staring at the sky. A surprising number of pedestrians stopped and began staring at the sky in conformity with the actors.

Asch Experiment – Conformity Bias

Solomon Asch gathered 123 college-aged subjects in an alleged test of visual perception. He assigned each subject to a group with 7 to 9 other persons, all of whom, unknown to the subject, were confederates of the investigator.

The investigator presented each group with 2 cards. One was a reference card with 3 vertical lines of obviously differing lengths. The other was a test card with 1 vertical line equal in length to one of the 3 lines on the reference card. He went around each group asking the members to call out the reference line to which the test line was equal in length. Asch arranged the groups such that the subject was always the last to give an answer. As a control, the subjects were also tested alone.

Each group had 3 trials, with a different pair of cards on each trial. The confederates were told in advance to give the correct answer on the first two trials but the same wrong answer on the third trial.

The results were that when tested alone, the subjects gave a wrong answer 1% of the time. However, in the groups, the subjects gave the wrong answer 36.8% of the time (Asch 1955).

Medical Examples of the Conformity Bias

Examples of the conformity bias in medicine are familiar and unfortunate. The problems include the Dalkon Shield, Vioxx, the past conditions at Walter Reed Army Medical Center, and the Tuskegee Experiment, among others. In each of these cases, numerous individuals conformed to the group regarding inappropriate policies and patterns when they actually knew better.

The conformity bias can be "weaponized" for purposes of manipulation. Many years ago, in a relatively rare occurrence, a pharmaceutical representative visited the author's office. These "drug reps" or "detail people" often develop background information on a physician's prescribing before visiting the physician's office! The "drug rep" indicated he was aware the author seldom prescribed oxycodone. The already irritated author replied that there was only rare need for it in the practice.

Initially appearing to change the topic, the drug rep asked if any of the author's patients were in physical therapy. When the author acknowledged that some were, he proceeded to impart the "information" that "physical therapy hurts" and that the other doctors were prescribing oxycodone for their patients in physical therapy! His attempt to "weaponize" the conformity bias did not change the author's prescribing philosophy.

The conformity bias is especially dangerous in medicine for three reasons: First, the consequences may be life or death. Second, the *independent* opinions of well-qualified authorities are critical. Third, the conformity bias seems to eventuate in decisions more extreme than the decisions of the same persons acting as individuals (Lamm and Myers 1978).

Countermeasure to Conformity Bias

A simple and decisive countermeasure to the conformity bias is to **focus on the decision being made and to ignore the simultaneous decisions of others**. This is the method Dr. James Lock described to Dr. Jerome Groopman when he said, "When a case first arrives, I don't want to hear anyone else's diagnosis. I look at the primary data" (Groopman 2008, p. 146). As indicated previously, this is also an effective countermeasure against the availability and confirmation biases.

Conclusion

The conformity bias militates against the very purpose of soliciting multiple inputs. The advantage of multiple inputs is that biases in various directions average out and that gaps in knowledge compensate for one another (Novella 2012, p. 184; Surowiecki 2014, p. 124). Consequently, relative attenuation of the effects of bias occurs only when the opinions forming the consensus are truly independent. Independence of component opinions is paramount.

References

Asch, S. E. (n.d.). Asch Conformity Task. *PsycTESTS Dataset.* doi:10.1037/t31951-000Solomon Asch

Asch, S. E. (1955). Opinions and Social Pressure. *Scientific American, 193*(5), 31-35. doi:10.1038/scientificamerican1155-31

Lamm, H., & Myers, D. G. (1978). Group-Induced Polarization of Attitudes and Behavior. *Advances in Experimental Social Psychology,* 145-195. doi:10.1016/s0065-2601(08)60007-6

Novella, S. (2012). *Your Deceptive Mind.* Lecture. The Great Courses.

Surowiecki, J. (2014). *The wisdom of crowds why the many are smarter than the few.* London: Abacus.

Chapter 9: Diffusion of Responsibility

Diffusion of Responsibility

Diffusion of responsibility is a phenomenon in which persons in groups are less likely to take responsibility than persons alone. Diffusion of responsibility is sometimes considered an attribution bias in that all parties involved attribute responsibility to someone else.

Darley-Latane Experiment 1

In 1964, 28-year-old Kitty Genovese was stabbed to death outside her apartment building in Queens, New York City. The attack was reported in the *New York Times* as having lasted over half an hour and having been seen or heard by 37 witnesses who did not call police.

The inaction of witnesses attracted the attention of many, including psychologists John Darley and Bibb Latane, who devised this experiment.

Darley and Latane recruited as subjects New York University undergraduates and told them they would participate in a discussion of how students adjust to university life. The subjects were told that to reduce embarrassment the discussion participants would be in separate rooms communicating by intercom and that the intercom would allow only one student to speak at a time for two minutes, after which it would switch to the next student.

The subjects were divided into three groups. Group 1 subjects were told that there would be one other person in the discussion. Group 2 subjects were told that there would be two. Group 3 subjects were told that there would be five. In reality, the subject was the only legitimate discussion participant; another "participant" was a confederate; and, the other voices, if any, were recordings.

During the first round of the discussion, the confederate indicated that at first he had difficulties concentrating on studies. He then added that sometimes he had severe seizures when under stress.

During the confederate's second turn to speak, he began normally, and then he began sounding in trouble, saying,

"I-er-um I think I-I need-er-if-if could er-er somebody er-er-er-er-er-er give me a little help here because-er-I-er-I'm-er-h-h-having a-a-a real problem-er right now and I-er-if somebody could help me out it would-it would-er-er-er s-s-sure be good ... because-er-there-er-ag cause I er-I-uh-I've got one of the-er-sei-er-er-things coming on and-and-and I could really use some help so if somebody would-er give me a little h-help-uh-er-er-er-er c-could somebody-er er-help-er-uh-uh-uh [choking sounds] ... I'm gonna die-er-er ... help-er-er-seizure [chokes, then quiet]."

The results of the experiment were that when the subject believed there was one other person in the group, 80% helped; when he/she believed there were two others in the group, 50% helped; when he/she believed there were five others in the group, 30% helped.

Finally, reminiscent of the Kitty Genovese case, when the subject believed there was one other person in the group, 100% reported the emergency; when he/she believed there were two others in the group, 85% reported; when he/she believed there were five other in the group, 60% reported (Darley 1968).

Darley-Latane Experiment 2

Darley, Latane, and Siegal, in 1968, recruited psychology students to participate in interviews to "discuss some of the problems involved in life at an urban university." On arrival, the students were asked to sit in a waiting room and complete a preliminary questionnaire. After a few minutes, smoke began to enter the room through a vent. The smoke intensified until visibility in the room was impaired.

Some of the students were in the waiting room alone. Others were in the waiting room with two or three other "interviewees," who were actually confederates, coached to act passively in the situation.

The results were that 55% of the subjects who were alone reported the smoke within two minutes, while only 12% of the subjects in the other two groups did so. After four minutes, 75% of the solitary subjects had reported the smoke while no additional subjects in the other two groups reported it (Siegal 1972).

Countermeasures to Diffusion of Responsibility

The best ways of avoiding diffusion of responsibility seem to be
   • Keep the group small.
   • Sharply define the identity and responsibilities of each member of the group.
   • Define those responsibilities in a *relevant* measurable way.
   • Frequently review performance of each member as revealed by those measurements.

- Provide feedback to each member of the group about their performance on a regular schedule.
- Establish a well-defined and clearly articulated program to remediate minor shortcomings.

Diffusion of Responsibility in Medicine

Diffusion of responsibility is becoming an increasing concern in medicine. At one time, patients had their family physician for life, or at least for a very long time. Aside from an occasional surgical referral, there were very few "hand offs" to other physicians.

Today's situation is dramatically different. Many physicians are employed and seek a new opportunity every few years. Those remaining with the same employer may be reassigned to a different office. Patients may switch physicians frequently as their insurance changes. Patients increasingly seek primary care in the emergency department or urgent care facilities. Increasingly, patients are switched upon inpatient admission from their primary care physician to a hospitalist, and back again upon discharge. Increasing numbers of subspecialists are becoming involved in the patient's care. Even in the primary care office, patients are subjected to multiple professionals. The medical "team" is growing larger and larger and the number of patient "handoffs" is increasing dramatically.

It is time to look critically upon the current care model. Seeking "warm handoffs" is okay; but the best way to address a problem is not to have it. Perhaps it is time to consider reducing the size of the group and diminishing the number of handoffs. The production-line model may have worked well for model-T Fords but may not work well for our patients.

Further, it is important to define the identity and responsibilities of each team member, including the team leader, and to communicate those responsibilities to the patient. It may be convenient for the team leader to abdicate responsibility and it may be humbling for other members to admit that they report to someone else; however, clear definitions of responsibility can reduce errors and better serve the patient.

Moreover, the satisfaction of those responsibilities should be measured in a *relevant* way, i.e., in a way related to clinical outcomes with patients. The metric used to measure the satisfaction of these well-defined responsibilities should be kept separate from any other metrics, especially those regarding productivity.

Conclusion

Diffusion of responsibility is a well-documented and studied phenomenon. Like other biases, it is a tendency to act that often lies below the level of attention. Periodic exhortations not to be a "slacker" are not sufficient to deal with the problem. Satisfactory countermeasures must be implemented especially with the increasing impact of the problem upon medical care.

References

Darley, J. M., & Latane, B. (1968). Bystander intervention in emergencies: Diffusion of responsibility. Journal of Personality and Social Psychology,8(4, Pt.1), 377-383. doi:10.1037/h0025589

Nisbett, R. E., & Borgida, E. (1975). Attribution and the psychology of prediction. Journal of Personality and Social Psychology,32(5), 932-943. doi:10.1037//0022-3514.32.5.932

Siegal, H. A., Latane, B., & Darley, J. (1972). The Unresponsive Bystander: Why Doesnt He Help? Contemporary Sociology,1(3), 226. doi:10.2307/2063973

Further Reading

Darley, J. M., & Latane, B. (1968). Bystander intervention in emergencies: Diffusion of responsibility. Journal of Personality and Social Psychology,8(4, Pt.1), 377-383. doi:10.1037/h0025589

Chapter 10: Stanley Milgram and Authority Bias

Stanley Milgram's Experiment

In 1963, **Stanley Milgram** published one of psychology's most interesting and relevant experiments. Milgram was motivated by the "just following orders" defense embraced by Nazi war criminals.

Milgram's Experiment

Milgram's subjects consisted of 40 males between ages 20 and 50 from the New Haven area. The subjects were of all educational levels from grade school to doctorate and believed they were participating in an experiment to determine "how much punishment is best for learning." The subjects received payment of $4.50 just for appearing at the lab.

Two "subjects" were led to a well-appointed lab on the Yale campus; but one of the "subjects" was a confederate in the experiment. They were introduced to a 31-year-old male experimenter in a gray technician's coat. The "true" subject was told to select a slip from a hat to determine if he were to be "teacher" or "learner." However, all the slips read "teacher" and the confederate dutifully accepted his role as "learner."

Teacher and learner were then led to an adjacent room where the learner was placed into an "electric chair" device and restrained with straps "to prevent excessive movement" while he was being shocked. The experimenter then applied an electrode to the learner's wrist "to avoid blisters and burns" and told the teacher, "Although the shocks can be extremely painful, they cause no permanent tissue damage."

The teacher was then led to an authentic looking instrument panel with an engraved plate reading "Shock Generator, Type ZLB, Dyson Instrument Company, Waltham, Mass. Output 15 Volts – 450 Volts." The "shock generator" had 30 switches, marked in 15-volt increments from 15 volts to 450 volts. Under each set of four switches was a label, reading progressively, "Slight Shock," "Moderate Shock," "Strong Shock," "Very Strong Shock," "Intense Shock," "Extreme Intensity Shock," "Danger: Severe Shock," and, under the last two switches, "XXX."

The teacher was then given a sample shock by having an electrode attached to his wrist while the experimenter depressed the 45-volt switch on the generator.

The teacher could not see that the 45-volt shock was actually delivered by a battery that bypassed the generator.

The teacher was then told that his role was to read a series of word pairs to the learner and then read the first word of the pair to the learner along with four terms. The learner was to indicate which of the four terms had originally been paired with the first word by flipping one of four switches that, in turn, would illuminate one of four lights on the teacher's console.

The experimenter instructed the teacher that each time the learner gave a wrong answer, the teacher was to move one level higher on the shock generator, announce the voltage, and then deliver the shock. The experimenter also had instructed the teacher to continue until the learner learned all the pairs correctly.

Meanwhile, the learner had a predetermined set of responses to the word-pair test, with approximately three wrong answers to one correct answer. At shock level 300 volts, the learner began pounding on the wall between the two rooms and stopped answering the questions. At this point, the experimenter instructed the teacher to treat the absence of a response as a wrong answer and to increase the shock level one step.

Whenever the teacher indicated that he did not wish to proceed, the experimenter instituted a standardized series of prods, thusly
- "Prod 1: Please continue."
- "Prod 2: The experiment requires that you continue."
- "Prod 3: It is absolutely essential that you continue."
- "Prod 4: You have no other choice, you *must* go on."

The series of prods began anew each time the teacher showed reluctance to follow orders. If the teacher refused to obey the experimenter after Prod 4, the experiment was terminated.

If the teacher said that the learner did not want to go on, the experimenter replied, "Whether the learner likes it or not, you must go on until he has learned all the word pairs correctly. So please go on." [This was followed by Prods 2, 3, and 4 if necessary.]

Milgram's Results

Milgram's results were astounding. **Despite the learner's pounding and kicking the wall between the two rooms, 26 of the 40 subjects were "obedient" to authority, continuing the experiment to the maximum level of 450 supposed volts.**

Five stopped at 300 volts, four at 315 volts, two at 330 volts, one at 345 volts, one at 360 volts, four at 375 volts, two at 390 volts, one at 405 volts, and one at 420 volts, for a total of 14 "defiant" of authority (Milgram 1963).

Conclusion

The Milgram experiment has been repeated many times and in many cultures. While the proportions of "obedient" and "defiant" subjects varied, all iterations of the experiment demonstrated the extreme pervasiveness of the bias of obedience to authority.

Having thus considered Milgram's demonstration of the presence and strength of authority as a psychological bias, it is time now to investigate appeal to authority as a logical fallacy.

Appeal to Authority as Logical Fallacy

Appeal to authority is common in daily life and medical practice. Physicians regularly refer patients to specialists or subspecialists for consultation and/or management. While appeal to authority is, to some degree, fraught by danger, it is unavoidable as one cannot, on their own, be an expert in all things at all times. Fortunately, **criteria exist to suggest when reliance on authority is more likely to be appropriate**.

Identifiable and Accessible Authority

First, the authority should be identifiable and accessible. Otherwise, the "authority" may not even exist, or, may not have made the statements ascribed to him or her. Hearsay evidence is not admissible in court because the supposed witness is not able to take the stand and testify under cross-examination.

Further, experts can be wrong. They should be identifiable and accessible to explain and defend their opinion or assertions as well as their qualifications to hold that opinion or make those assertions.

Occasionally, one hears verbal vague attributions such as "a famous scientist," or "someone," or "a friend of a friend." More frequently, one sees unspecified authorities invoked in written text as assertions without supporting footnotes. Sometimes, vague citations of authority are made such as "as seen on TV." Finally, inappropriate citations of authority are made such as "because it is not on The Formulary" or "because it is the Policy of the XYZ Health System."

Relevant Authority

Second, the "authority" should actually be an authority in the area in which he or she presents evidence.

While totally unrelated authorities are rarely presented, sports figures are sometimes presented advertising breakfast cereals on the tenuous supposition that because they perform well in sports, they must be knowledgeable in nutrition.

Similarly, athletes are featured in advertisements for patent medications related to muscular strains and sprains. Here the tenuous supposition is that they must frequently be injured and therefore must be expert in medications for strains and sprains.

Astoundingly, actors in hospital dramas appear in television commercials advertising patent medications and citing as their authority that they "play a doctor on TV" (I'm not a Doctor, but I play one on TV, 1986).

Testimonials feature inappropriate authorities. Here, patients or patient's family members are presented as true experts on the treatment of a disease.

Finally, references may be made to a journal in order to invoke as an authority the journal's "brand" or to invoke as an authority proximity to academic articles in the journal. The reference is sometimes only to an advertisement in the journal.

Unbiased Authority

Third, the authority should be unbiased and without the prospect of profit from delivered statements or opinions. The problem of biased authority breaks down into situations in which the presence of bias is known and situations in which the presence of bias is unknown.

Biased Standards of Care

An authority that is both compelling and impersonal is the "standard of care." The fact that standards of care are impersonal authorities conduces to the impression that they are objective. This is not necessarily the case.

Two biased standards to be examined here are "custom" and "deferred decision."

Custom as a Biased Standard

In the past, industry custom played an important part in determining legally accepted performance standards. Nevertheless, customs as a standard of care periodically need to be updated, and, at that point, are subject to many biases. Among these are the availability bias, the bandwagon effect, the confirmation bias, the endowment effect, and, most conspicuously, what psychologists today would call, the *status quo* bias.

Custom as a standard of care began changing with the *T. J. Hooper* Case of 1932.

T. J. Hooper Case

The *T. J. Hooper* was a tugboat towing two coal barges up the east coast of the US. It ran afoul of bad weather off New Jersey and lost the coal barges. The owner of the coal sued the owners of the *T. J. Hooper*, claiming that the loss was the result of negligence since the *Hooper* did not have the newly emerging technology of radio for the reception of weather forecasts. The *Hooper*'s owners argued no negligence since radio receivers were not (yet) the industry custom.

Judge Learned Hand ruled that custom is not dispositive of what the reasonable person will do. He continued, "A whole calling may have unduly lagged in the adoption of new and available devices. It never may set its own tests, however persuasive be its usages"(Cheng 2017). Judge Hand further stated, "There are precautions so imperative that even their universal disregard will not excuse their omission" (Helling n.d.)

Nevertheless, medicine lagged behind other areas and retained custom as a standard of care until the 1974 case of Helling v. Carey (Moffett 2011).

Helling v. Carey Case

Plaintiff Barbara Helling was a 32-year-old female who had initially seen ophthalmologists, Dr. Thomas Carey and Dr. Robert Laughlin in 1959 for contact lenses. In 1963, she began complaining of eye irritation possibly caused by the contact lenses and saw the ophthalmologists 10 times from 1963 until 1968. However, Helling actually had open-angle glaucoma, which was not diagnosed by the doctors until they measured eye pressure (tonometry) at her 10th appointment with them in October 1968.

Helling sued the ophthalmologists, alleging that negligence on their part for not measuring her eye pressure caused her permanent vision loss. At trial, expert witnesses testified that the standards of the specialty did not require tonometry for patients less than 40 years of age (Helling 2017). The Trial Court and Appeals Court accepted this argument.

However, the Supreme Court of the State of Washington overruled the lower courts and found the defendants negligent. The Supreme Court found, "A greater duty of care could be imposed on the defendants than was established by their profession," and "the reasonable standard that should have been followed under the undisputed facts of this case was the timely giving of this simple, harmless pressure test" (Helling n.d.).

In rendering its decision, the Supreme Court also referenced the *T. J. Hooper* Case and quoted Oliver Wendell Holmes 1903 statement, "What usually is done may be evidence of what ought to be done, but what ought to be done is fixed by a standard of reasonable prudence, whether it usually is complied with or not."

The Helling vs. Carey decision heralded the beginning of a **transition from "custom" as the standard of care in medicine to the "reasonable and prudent physician" as the standard of care.**

Deferred Decision as a Biased Standard

The formulation of standards can be a daunting task. No wonder it is frequently avoided with the argument that the situations the standards are intended to address are too complicated to be anticipated and that the individuals in the situation have the best knowledge of the problem and shouldn't be constrained in their options.

However, the fact is that *a priori* standards are implemented in order to foster consistent, enlightened decision-making and diminish bias by addressing the problem before the fact, in a situation in which the biases are absent or reduced. **To systematically defer the decision to the developing situation is to abrogate standards and increase the effect of biases.**

At a recent medical meeting attended by the author, a debate erupted regarding exact supervisory standards for physicians with respect to mid-level professionals. Some of the physicians in attendance adopted the position that the decision should be left to those in the situation, in their words, "at the practice level." Nevertheless, this defers the determination of standards to those with a substantial and immediate conflict of interest. A deferred determination of standards cannot help being a biased determination of standards.

Inadequate Ability to Compensate for *Known* Biased Authority

Many physicians believe that they can allow for known bias in those presenting them with information, but evidence shows otherwise (Goldacre 2014, p 274). This inability is consistent with the bias-blind-spot bias discussed in Chapter 5.

The inability to compensate for known bias is reminiscent of the non-sober alcoholic's allegation of being able to drink heavily because of being able to tolerate alcohol.

Steinman Study

Steinman's study provided significant evidence that **physicians overestimate their ability to allow for known bias in supplied information**.

Steinman surveyed 117 medical residents at a university-based internal medicine residency program in regard to the influence of pharmaceutical industry promotions upon physicians. Of the 117 residents, 105 completed the survey. Of these 105, 61% stated that industry promotions and contacts did not influence their own prescribing, but only 16% believed other physicians were similarly unaffected (Steinman 2001).

Orlowski Study

Further evidence of physician susceptibility to even obvious bias is supplied by Orlowski's study (Orlowski 1992). Orlowski followed the prescribing practices of two groups of 10 physicians each. The physicians were invited to all-expenses-paid trips to Sunbelt vacation sites to attend pharmaceutical company sponsored symposia. The drugs featured in each symposium were intravenous drugs used only in hospitalized patients.

Orlowski followed the usage patterns of the two drugs for 22 months preceding, and 17 months following each symposium. The prescribing of one drug increased from a mean of 81 +/- 44 units before the symposium to 272 +/- 117 units after. The prescribing of the other drug increased from a mean of 34 +/- 30 units before the symposium to 87 +/- 24 units after.

Conspicuously, 9 of the 10 physicians in the one group and 8 of the 10 in the other group insisted that such a trip would in no way influence their prescribing decisions.

Inadequate Ability to Compensate for *Unknown* Biased Authority

Certainly, the authority whose bias is unknown is more formidable than the authority whose bias is known. It is for this reason that the **presence of bias or monetary influence is sometimes deliberately made difficult to ascertain**.

Co-opting Patient Advocacy Organizations

Patient advocacy organizations are non-profit organizations of lay and professional persons dedicated to combating a particular disease or disability. Examples of the more prominent of these are the American Heart Association, the Arthritis Foundation, and the American Diabetes Association.

Patient advocacy organizations are at risk for being co-opted by for-profit health industries. They have the aura of credibility and authority in the disease area for which they advocate; this aura is coveted by for-profit health industries. Additionally, they also have the vulnerability of a constant need of finances to continue their activities, a need the for-profit health industries can readily fill.

Specifically, it is helpful to drug and device manufacturers for patient advocacy organizations to advocate for expediting to market the industries' drugs and treatments, even when such might not be in the best interest of patient safety. It is also helpful to for-profit industry for patient advocacy organizations to advocate for the government's paying for the industry's more expensive drugs and treatments when competitive and more economical alternatives are already available.

Rose Study

The Rose study compiled significant information on potentially compromised patient advocacy organizations (Rose 2013).

Rose cited the following data from Marshall and Aldous (Marshall 2006) on the percentage of total funding of various patient advocacy organizations obtained from pharmaceutical companies.
- Depression and Bipolar Support Alliance .... >50%
- Colorectal Cancer Coalition 80%
- Restless Legs Syndrome Foundation 44%
- Children and Adults with ADHD 22%
- Narcolepsy Network 35%
- Breast Cancer Action (does not accept company donations) 0%

Rose further cited the New York Times report (Harris 2009) on the National Alliance on Mental Illness (NAMI) indicating that from 2006 to 2008, drug makers contributed about three-quarters of all NAMI's donations. This was from the investigations by Senator Charles Grassley and from documents obtained by *The New York Times*.

NAMI, in response to the investigation, then began posting on its web site the names of companies donating $5000 or more. Senator Grassley subsequently praised NAMI for this disclosure.

McCoy Study

McCoy and colleagues studied potential conflicts of interest in patient advocacy organizations having substantial industry involvement (McCoy 2017). All the organizations had annual revenues of $7.5 million or more.

The McCoy group found that of 104 US-based patient advocacy organizations, 83% received financial support from drug, device, and biotechnology companies and that at least 39% had a current or former industry executive on their governing board. Moreover, 12% of the advocacy organizations had a current or former industry executive in a leadership position on the board.

Further, of the 104 patient advocacy organizations, only 60 listed the names of donors on their web site, only 23 listed the amounts of individual donations on their website, and only 8 listed the total revenue from industrial or corporate donations on their website.

Prasad Study

Prasad and Abola studied 68 cancer-patient advocacy organizations. Of these, 51 disclosed biopharmaceutical sponsorship. Interestingly, 16 did not respond, and only one specifically reported that it does not accept money from the biopharmaceutical industry (Abola 2016).

Countermeasures to Authority Bias

Several countermeasures to the authority bias appear above. They consist in **using only identifiable and accessible authorities, relevant authorities, and unbiased authorities**. Unidentifiable or inaccessible authorities constitute only hearsay evidence. Irrelevant authorities are, essentially, no authorities. Finally, biased authorities may be conveyors of disinformation.

Conclusion

Milgram demonstrated the powerful influence of the authority bias. Nevertheless, reliance on authority is sometimes unavoidable. When this is the case, the authority should be identifiable and accessible, relevant to the problem being addressed, and, as far as determinable, unbiased.

The ability to allow for known biases in authority is typically overestimated; the ability to allow for unknown biases in authority is likely even more compromised.

The "custom" standard is a highly biased standard falling into disrepute. It has largely been supplanted by the "reasonable and prudent physician" standard. The "deferred decision" standard is virtually no standard at all.

References

Abola, M. V., & Prasad, V. (2016). Industry Funding of Cancer Patient Advocacy Organizations. *Mayo Clinic Proceedings, 91*(11), 1668-1670. doi:10.1016/j.mayocp.2016.08.015

Cheng, E. K. (2017). *Rules versus Standards of Care*. Lecture. Lecture 4 in Torts in Law School for Everyone, The Great Courses, The Teaching Company, 2017.

Goldacre, B. (2014). Bad pharma: how drug companies mislead doctors and harm patients. New York: Faber & Faber, Inc., an affiliate of Farrar, Straus and Giroux.

Harris, G. (2009, October 21). Drug Makers Are Advocacy Group's Biggest Donors. *New York Times*.

Helling v. Carey Case Brief - Quimbee. (2017). Retrieved November 15, 2017, from https://www.bing.com/cr?IG=5C28386C82E748E8980038A1872E7F3D&CID=2AA31B2D64DF69593822101665D968A2&rd=1&h=-QjHIbiTaZVoDIarHJ0fdaP-4v9hlEX83fr6I8D9qNU&v=1&r=https%3a%2f%2fwww.quimbee.com%2fcases%2fhelling-v-carey&p=DevEx,5097.1

Helling v. Carey, 519 P.2d 981, 83 Wash. 2d 514 – CourtListener.com. (n.d.). Retrieved November 15, 2017, from https://www.courtlistener.com/opinion/1180369/helling-v-carey/

I'm not a Doctor, but I play one on TV Commercial 1986 with Peter Bergman Vicks Formula 44. (2012, February 03). Retrieved from https://youtu.be/ts0XG6qDIco

Marshall, J., & Aldhous, P. (2006). Swallowing the best advice? *New Scientist, 192*(2575), 18-22. doi:10.1016/s0262-4079(06)60831-2

Mccoy, M. S., Carniol, M., Chockley, K., Urwin, J. W., Emanuel, E. J., & Schmidt, H. (2017). Conflicts of Interest for Patient-Advocacy Organizations. *New England Journal of Medicine,376*(9), 880-885. doi:10.1056/nejmsr1610625

Milgram, S. (1963). Behavioral Study of obedience. *The Journal of Abnormal and Social Psychology,67*(4), 371-378. doi:10.1037/h0040525

Moffett, P., & Moore, G. (2011). The Standard of Care: Legal History and Definitions: the Bad and Good News. *West J Emerg Med, 12*(1), 109-112. Retrieved November 15, 2017.

Orlowski, J. P., & Wateska, L. (1992). The Effects of Pharmaceutical Firm Enticements on Physician Prescribing Patterns. *Chest, 102*(1), 270-273. doi:10.1378/chest.102.1.270

Rose, S. L. (2013). Patient Advocacy Organizations: Institutional Conflicts of Interest, Trust, and Trustworthiness. *The Journal of Law, Medicine & Ethics, 41*(3), 680-687. doi:10.1111/jlme.12078

Steinman, M. A., Shlipak, M. G., & Mcphee, S. J. (2001). Of principles and pens: attitudes and practices of medicine housestaff toward pharmaceutical industry promotions. *The American Journal of Medicine, 110*(7), 551-557. doi:10.1016/s0002-9343(01)00660-x

Further Reading

Goldacre, B. (2014). Bad pharma: how drug companies mislead doctors and harm patients. New York: Faber & Faber, Inc., an affiliate of Farrar, Straus and Giroux.

Milgram, S. (1963). Behavioral Study of obedience. *The Journal of Abnormal and Social Psychology,67*(4), 371-378. doi:10.1037/h0040525

Chapter 11: Framing Effect Bias

Framing Effect Bias

Framing effect bias is a tendency to make a decision based upon *circumstances surrounding* the presented evidence more than upon the evidence itself. Incredibly, a **preference between options can actually reverse with changes of frame** (Tversky and Kahneman 1981).

Common Example of the Framing Effect Bias

Credit card companies in the late 1970s insisted their affiliated merchants sign agreements prohibiting the merchants from passing along costs by charging a fee for payments by credit card. A bill, heavily opposed by the credit card companies, was introduced in Congress to prohibit such agreements. When it became obvious that some sort of bill would pass, the credit card companies retreated to a fallback position that any such bill should label prices as cash discounts rather than credit card surcharges. They obviously considered that fewer consumers would avoid credit card purchases if they forwent a cash discount instead of submitting to an equal credit card surcharge (Thaler 1980).

Tversky-Kahneman "Asian Disease" Experiment – Framing Bias

Tversky and Kahneman's subjects were 152 students from Stanford University and the University of British Columbia. The researchers presented the subjects with the scenario that an unusual Asian disease is expected to kill 600 people in the US. However, if program A is adopted, 200 people will be saved. On the other hand, if program B is adopted, there is a one-third probability that 600 people will be saved and a two-thirds probability that no people will be saved. Given a choice between the programs, 72% of the subjects chose program A and 28% chose program B.

Subjects in the experiment were students from Stanford University and the University of British Columbia. Tversky and Kahneman presented 152 subjects with the scenario that an unusual Asian disease is expected to kill 600 people in the US. However, if program A is adopted, 200 people will be saved. On the other hand, if program B is adopted, there is a one-third probability that 600 people will be saved and a two-thirds probability that no people will be saved. The results were that 72% of the subjects chose program A and 28% chose program B.

Next, the researchers presented 155 subjects with a similar scenario under different wording. They stated that if program C is adopted, 400 people will die, while if program D is adopted, there is a one-third probability that no one will die and a two-thirds probability that 600 people will die. The results this time were that 22% of subjects chose program C while 78% chose program D.

Here the equivalent A-C programs shifted from an endorsement of 72% down to 22% while the equivalent B-D programs shifted from an endorsement of 28% up to 78%, all predicated upon the wording of the scenario (Tversky and Kahneman 1981).

Medical Example and Tversky Experiment -- Framing Bias

In 1981, Tversky and colleagues published a study in which they assembled a large group of subjects none of whom was known to have lung cancer. The group was comprised of 238 men who were chronic medical patients, 424 radiologists, and 491 business school graduate students.

The researchers presented the subjects with a hypothetical scenario for lung cancer treatment involving surgery versus radiation. When the data were presented in terms of probability of mortality, radiation was preferred to surgery 42% of the time. When the same data were presented in terms of probability of survival, radiation was preferred 25% of the time.

Importantly, the general pattern of preferences was similar in all three groups (Tversky and Kahneman 1981). This result suggests that physicians should have no expectation of immunity against the framing effect because of their training.

Medical Example and Slovic Experiment – Framing Bias

Slovic and colleagues presented to experienced psychologists and psychiatrists the scenario of making a discharge decision regarding a hospitalized psychiatric patient with a history of violence.

The experimenters presented the subject psychologists and psychiatrists with data in a natural frequency format, namely, that 10 in 100 patients with a similar history committed violence against others within six months of discharge. With this format, 41% opposed discharge.

The experimenters also presented the subject psychologists and psychiatrists with the equivalent data but in a probability format, namely, that determined from patients with a similar history, there was a 10% probability of the patient committing violence against others within six months of discharge. In this case, only 21% opposed discharge.

The substantial influence of the framing bias must be respected when such a simple change in the presentation of a scenario can so significantly alter critical decisions made by educated and experienced professionals.

Countermeasures to the Framing Bias

Although the framing bias is powerful, some countermeasures are available.

First, if the information can be obtained independently, it may be possible to bypass sources biasedly framing the information.

Second, it may be possible to reframe the information oneself (Huettel 2014). This is easily accomplished in the two examples above citing the Tversky experiments.

Third, a powerful countermeasure exists in the use of natural frequencies instead of probabilities. The **natural frequency phraseology presents a clearer representation of the data** useful to the physician both for the solution of problems and the explanation of options to the patient (Gigerenzer 2015, p. 126, 169; Goldacre 2010, p. 187).

Conclusion

It is tempting and self-assuring to assume that intelligent people make decisions based upon evidence and not upon the manner in which the evidence is expressed. Unfortunately, much evidence from experimental psychology suggests that this is not so and that framing the evidence affects the direction of decisions made by both the general public and medical professionals.

References

Gigerenzer, G. (2015). *Risk savvy: how to make good decisions*. London: Penguin Books.

Goldacre, B. (2010). Bad science: quacks, hacks and big pharma -- flacks --. New York: Faber and Faber.

Huettel, S. (2014). Framing - Moving to a Different Perspective. Lecture. In Behavioral Economics: When Psychology and Economics Collide (pp. 158-164). The Great Courses.

Kahneman, D., & Tversky, A. (1984). Choices, values, and frames. American Psychologist,39(4), 341-350. doi:10.1037/0003-066x.39.4.341

McNeil, B. J., Pauker, S. G., Sox, H. C., & Tversky, A. (1982). On the Elicitation of Preferences for Alternative Therapies. New England Journal of Medicine,306(21), 1259-1262. doi:10.1056/nejm198205273062103

Slovic, P., Monahan, J., & Macgregor, D. G. (2000). Patient Violence Risk Measure. PsycTESTS Dataset. doi:10.1037/t38088-000

Further Reading

Gigerenzer, G. (2015). *Risk savvy: how to make good decisions*. London: Penguin Books.
Goldacre, B. (2010). Bad science: quacks, hacks and big pharma -- flacks --. New York: Faber and Faber.

Chapter 12: Novelty Bias, Halo Effect, and Information Bias

This chapter presents the novelty bias, halo effect, and information bias. These all contribute to bad decision-making by replacing relevant information with irrelevant information.

Novelty Bias

Novelty is both a **cognitive bias** and a **logical fallacy**.

As a **logical fallacy**, it is a subcase of affirming the consequent (see Chapter 15). It mistakenly concludes that since improvements on an initial idea, invention, procedure, or medication are newer than the initial idea or invention, that therefore whatever is newer must be an improvement.

As a **cognitive bias**, it is a **systematic judgment, without evidence, below the level of attention, and tending to persist when resisted, that whatever is newer is better.**

Novelty here is considered predominantly as a cognitive bias.

Common Examples of Novelty Bias

The novelty bias circumvents rationality and overwhelms the advice to "contain the damage" whenever one determines to implement any new plan under the rationale that it will be better than the current system.

One pays the price of the novelty bias each time one **downloads and installs, without any evidence of potential improvement, the latest version of a program or operating system**, only to find that some of the most needed applications no longer operate under the "upgrade."

Medical Example of Novelty Bias

In 1936, the Food, Drug, and Cosmetic (FD&C) Act became law and ensured that medications were safe. In 1962, The FD&C Act was strengthened by the Kefauver-Harris Amendment to insure that medications were not just safe, but that they actually worked. The 1962 act had in its provisions that drugs brought onto the market between 1936 and 1962 were to be evaluated retroactively for evidence that those drugs actually worked.

The result of the Kefauver-Harris Amendment was that **600 drugs, marketed from 1936 to 1962, were withdrawn from the market because no proof existed that the newly introduced drugs were actually effective** (Green 2012).

Countermeasures to the Novelty Bias

Countermeasures to the novelty bias consist in challenging both the proposal's novelty and its effectiveness.

It is often helpful, in considering a proffered proposal, to ask the question **"How is this different from the present system or a past system?"** Sometimes, this question has a legitimate answer; it may be that advances in technology are allowing for improved implementation of a present or past system. Sometimes, however, the "novelty" is just window dressing.

Another helpful countermeasure is **to examine the evidence for effectiveness of the proposal**. A new but useless proposal is of no benefit.

Halo Effect

The "halo effect" is the **tendency to generalize one positive or negative trait or the overall impression of a person, thing, or situation to other traits, even traits of which nothing is known**. It is related to the confirmation bias and was first documented by Edward Thorndike in 1920 (Thorndike 1920).

Thorndike Study -- Halo Effect

In 1919, psychologist Walter Dill Scott created a rating plan for the selection of military aviators for the US Army Air Service. The plan listed separate categories for physical qualities, intelligence, leadership, and character. Scott specifically instructed those completing the rating to consider each of the four categories *independently*.

Nevertheless, when Edward Thorndike reviewed the completed evaluations, he found that apparently unrelated qualities, such as intelligence and physique, correlated in the ratings. He attributed this to systematic error on the part of the evaluators in that evaluations of intelligence influenced evaluations of physical qualities, despite instructions to the evaluators to keep them separate (Thorndike 1920).

Landy Experiment -- Halo Effect

In 1974, David Landy selected as subjects 60 male undergraduates and presented them with an essay supposedly written by a female college freshman. Of the 60 male undergraduates, 30 read a version of the essay that was well written and 30 read a version that was poorly written. In each group, 10 subjects were presented a picture of an attractive female as the purported author; 10 subjects were presented a picture of an unattractive female as the purported author; and, 10 subjects were presented no picture.

The subjects evaluated the well-written essay more favorably than the poorly written essay. However, they also rated the essay most well written when the purported author was attractive, least well written when the purported author was unattractive, and intermediately when no picture accompanied the essay (Landy 1974).

Common Examples -- Halo Effect

It is no accident that **advertisements typically show attractive people happily interacting with the promoted product**. This approach exploits the fact that attractiveness of a spokesperson or model engenders a positive perception of the featured item. An abundance of marketing and advertising research supports this technique (Baker 1977, Caballero 1989, Caballero 1984, Chaiken 1979). In the words of psychologist Karen Dion, "What is beautiful is good" (Dion 1972)

Medical Examples -- Halo Effect

Medical examples not only exemplify the halo effect, but, indeed, are its poster child. **Television commercials featuring attractive actors with smiling faces in pastoral surroundings convey a positive image of a promoted drug**, while a voice-over relates a litany of serious and sometimes fatal side effects (Kaplan Thaler Group, Lyrica TV Commercial ""Keep Moving"; McCann Erickson Agency, Viagra TV Commercial "Red Convertible"; Publicis North America Agency, Humira TV Commercial "Back in Shape"; Publicis North America Agency, Humira TV Commercial "Day at the Fair").

Nevertheless, the visual, emotional messages overwhelm the oral, factual ones; and, the ads persist because they are effective.

Countermeasures to the Halo Effect

As a countermeasure to the halo effect when selecting among options, it is important to keep a narrow focus and **avoid overall impressions**. Kahneman advises **identifying in advance the most important independent component factors and devising a simple rating system for them**. He then advises **scoring each factor before moving to the next**. He **cautions against returning and changing scores after proceeding to the next option** (Kahneman Page 232-233 of 512, Kindle location 3876-3892 of 9398).

This approach requires substantial discipline but provides a degree of isolation from the insidious halo effect.

Information Bias

Information bias is the tendency to seek further information when that information will not influence the decision being considered. Baron identified the bias in 1988 and felt that the bias was especially significant when information was costly as is the case in science, the professions, and commerce (Baron 1988). We emphasize that the bias is especially important in medicine where the acquisition of information can be physically dangerous.

Baron Experiment – Information Bias

In a complex 1988 experiment, Baron proposed to 33 subjects, all University of Pennsylvania undergraduate and graduate students, a fictitious patient with fictitious differential diagnoses in the following situation:

"A patient's presenting symptoms and history suggest a diagnosis of globoma, with about .8 probability. If it isn't globoma, it's either popitis or flapemia. Each disease has its own treatment, which is ineffective against the other two diseases. A test called the ET scan would certainly yield a positive result if the patient had popitis, and a negative result if she has flapemia. If the patient has globoma, positive and negative results are equally likely. If the ET scan were the only test you could do, should you do it? Why or why not?" (Baron 1988)

Here the **"ET scan" could not possibly change the course of action of the physician, who must consider "globoma" as the dominating differential diagnosis**.

However, Baron reports that although a majority of the 33 subjects answered correctly, interviews with those who were incorrect suggested that the information bias prevented them from understanding the relevance of certain information

(Baron 1988). These results are intriguing and certainly require replication and further development. If these results are corroborated, they will have substantial medical significance.

Medical Significance – Information Bias

The **tendency to pursue additional information when it will not change medical decision-making certainly wastes resources** that could better be used for prevention, education, public health, patient treatment, and research. However, there is an additional problem.

Unnecessary and irrelevant diagnostic tests carry risk in themselves. An estimated 510 people in every 100,000 are estimated to develop cancers other than leukemia from the ionizing radiation of CT scans (Costello 2013). Although this is small compared to the 19,800 of every 100,000 people who develop cancer without such diagnostic radiation, the fact remains that a portion of those 510 cases may be avoidable. Again, diagnostic endoscopies and biopsies carry risks in themselves, and so do the anesthetic procedures accompanying them. An additional problem resulting from this disconnected pursuit of information is that the **inappropriate studies ordered have intrinsic information errors, they report false positives**. The false positives then result in further tests or procedures that have their own costs and complications.

Particularly dangerous is the penetration of the information bias into public policy. This can occur with a program to institute screening procedures for conditions having a low base rate in the screened population. Here the number of false positives can dwarf the number of true positives and the morbidity and mortality from pursuing the false positives may exceed the morbidity and mortality from the screened-for disease. More follows on screening in Chapters 14 and 22.

Countermeasure to Information Bias

An effective countermeasure to the information bias consists in asking, **"How will this new information change the decision?"** If the new information will not change the decision, then the acquisition of new information is a waste of time, money, resources, and possibly a danger to the patient.

Conclusion

This chapter has discussed the novelty bias, the halo effect, and the information bias, all of which replace relevant information with irrelevant information in decision-making. The chapter has presented descriptions of these biases, along with their impact and countermeasures to them.

References

Asch, S. E. (1946). Forming impressions of personality. The Journal of Abnormal and Social Psychology,41(3), 258-290. doi:10.1037/h0055756

Baker, M. J., & Churchill, G. A. (1977). The Impact of Physically Attractive Models on Advertising Evaluations. Journal of Marketing Research,14(4), 538. doi:10.2307/3151194

Baron, J., Beattie, J., & Hershey, J. C. (1988). Heuristics and biases in diagnostic reasoning. Organizational Behavior and Human Decision Processes,42(1), 88-110. doi:10.1016/0749-5978(88)90021-0

Caballero, M. J., Lumpkin, J. R., & Madden, C. S. (august/september 1989). Using Physical Attractiveness as an Advertising Tool. Journal of Advertising Research,16-22. Retrieved June 19, 2017.

Caballero, M. J., & Solomon, P. J. (1984). Effects of Model Attractiveness on Sales Response. Journal of Advertising,13(1), 17-33. doi:10.1080/00913367.1984.10672870

Chaiken, S. (1979). Communicator physical attractiveness and persuasion. Journal of Personality and Social Psychology,37(8), 1387-1397. doi:10.1037//0022-3514.37.8.1387

Costello, J. E., Cecava, N. D., Tucker, J. E., & Bau, J. L. (2013). CT Radiation Dose: Current Controversies and Dose Reduction Strategies. American Journal of Roentgenology,201(6), 1283-1290. doi:10.2214/ajr.12.9720

Dion, K., Berscheid, E., & Walster, E. (1972). What is beautiful is good. Journal of Personality and Social Psychology,24(3), 285-290. doi:10.1037/h0033731

Emerson, G. B., Warme, W. J., Wolf, F. M., Heckman, J. D., Brand, R. A., & Leopold, S. S. (2010). Testing for the Presence of Positive-Outcome Bias in Peer Review. Archives of Internal Medicine,170(21). doi:10.1001/archinternmed.2010.406

Gonzalez, A. B., Mahesh, M., & Kim, K. (2010). Projected Cancer Risks from Computed Tomographic Scans Performed in the United States in 2007. Journal of Vascular Surgery,51(3), 783. doi:10.1016/j.jvs.2010.01.041

Greene, J. A., & Podolsky, S. H. (18 october 2012). Reform, Regulation, and Pharmaceuticals — The Kefauver–Harris Amendments at 50. New England Journal of Medicine,367(16), 1481-1483. doi:10.1056/nejmp1210007

Kahneman, D. (2015). *Thinking, fast and slow*. New York: Farrar, Straus and Giroux.

Landy, D., & Sigall, H. (1974). Beauty is talent: Task evaluation as a function of the performers physical attractiveness. Journal of Personality and Social Psychology,29(3), 299-304. doi:10.1037/h0036018

Leopold, S. S. (2010). Testing for the Presence of Positive-Outcome Bias in Peer Review

McCann Erickson Agency (Writer). (n.d.). Viagra TV Commercial "Red Convertible"[Television broadcast]. In Viagra TV Commercial "Red Convertible".

Publicis North America Agency (Writer). (n.d.). Humira TV Commercial "Day at the Fair"[Television broadcast]. In Humira TV Commercial "Day at the Fair". Kaplan Thaler Group (Writer). (n.d.). Lyrica TV Commercial "Moving More"[Television broadcast]. In Lyrica TV Commercial "Moving More".

Publicis North America Agency (Writer). (n.d.). Humira TV Commercial "Back in Shape"[Television broadcast]. In Humira TV Commercial "Back in Shape".

Thorndike, E. (1920). A constant error in psychological ratings. Journal of Applied Psychology,4(1), 25-29. doi:10.1037/h0071663

Further Reading

Kahneman, D. (2015). *Thinking, fast and slow*. New York: Farrar, Straus and Giroux.

Chapter 13: Search Satisfaction Bias

Search Satisfaction Bias

Search satisfaction bias is a tendency to prematurely terminate a search for abnormalities once an abnormality has been found (Gunderman 2009). It is exemplified in the emergency department dictum that the easiest fracture to miss is the *second* one. Radiology has produced a body of studies on the topic; however, the bias certainly affects other areas of medicine and of life.

Common Examples – Search Satisfaction Bias

Thieves take advantage of search satisfaction bias when they rob the same victim twice. Terrorists do the same when they plant two bombs at their target. Indeed, there are concerns that **finding a water bottle hidden in airport luggage might reduce the chances of security agents finding a box cutter** (Fleck 2010).

Fleck Experiments – Search Satisfaction Bias

In 2010, Mathias Fleck published 10 experiments to establish the first non-radiological existence of the search satisfaction bias. He used as subjects 30 Duke University undergraduates and exposed them to 250 trials. Each trial consisted of a 15-second view of a screen with 25 items.

Each item contained two perpendicular lines with the endpoint of line A being located at various locations along line B. Each screen had one, two, or three items with the endpoint of line A precisely at the center of line B, while all the others, the distractors, had the endpoint offset from the center (Fleck 2010, see Picture 13.1 below).

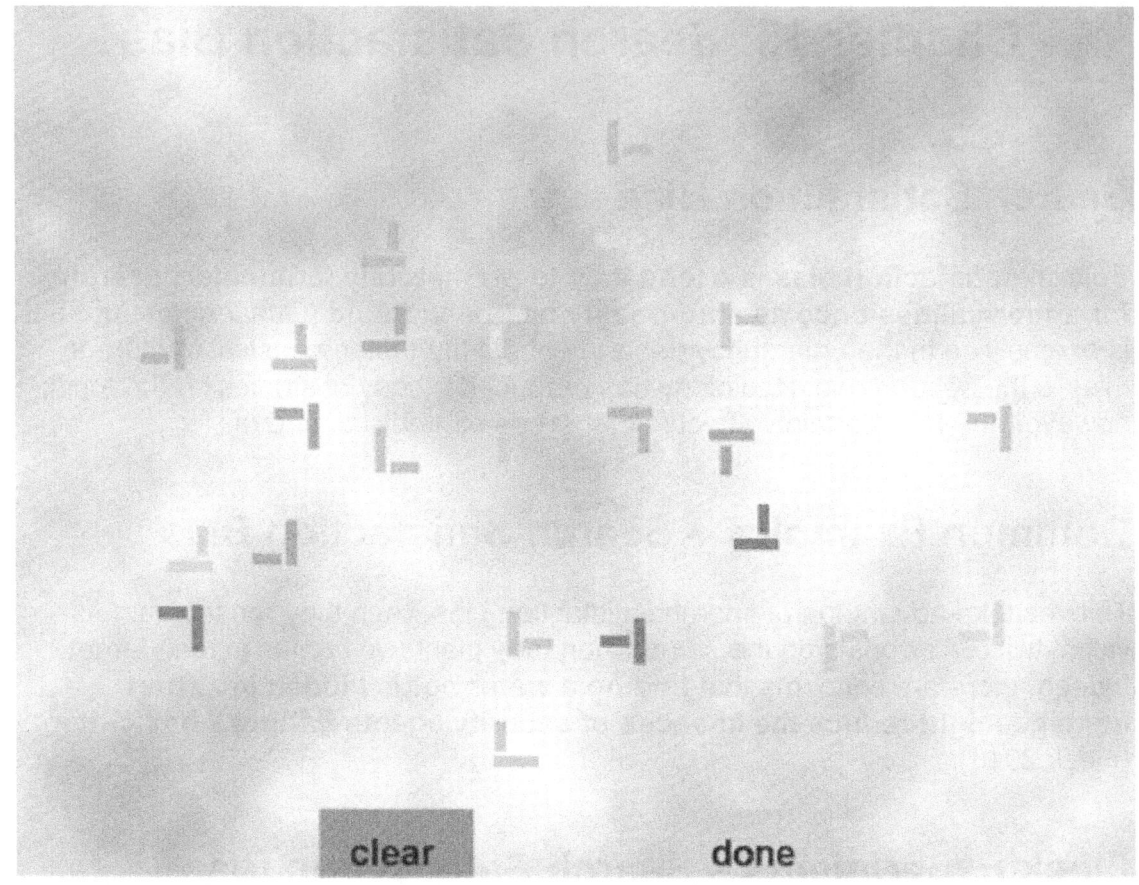

Picture 13.1 from "Generalized 'Satisfaction of Search': Adverse Influences on Dual-Target Search Accuracy" by Fleck, Samei, and Mitroff in *Journal of Experimental Psychology Applied*, March 2010

The task of the subjects was to identify these center-point perpendicularities within the 15 seconds.

Fleck's findings were
- As the ratio of the easily detected high-salience targets to the less easily detected low-salience targets increased, the subjects missed more low-salience targets. Search satisfaction increased.
- When the time limit increased to 30 seconds instead of 15 seconds, search satisfaction decreased.
- Even when rewards for accuracy incentivized subjects, search satisfaction occurred and increased under time pressure.
- Even when salience was eliminated and targets were perceptually identical, search satisfaction still occurred (Fleck 2010).

Medical Examples of Search Satisfaction Bias

Dr. Jerome Groopman reported the case of a 60-year-old woman described to him by Dr. Daniel Ginsberg. The patient presented with lower abdominal pain and urinary frequency. She briefly improved after antibiotics for urinary tract infection. Days later, her symptoms returned. A CT scan demonstrated a small mass in the right kidney and an enlarged appendix, considered by the radiologist to be a normal variant.

The patient underwent a laparoscopic right nephrectomy, but the surgery did not resolve her symptoms. She presented to the emergency room where she demonstrated a normal white blood cell count but with 82% neutrophils and elevated serum transaminases. Repeat CT scan showed a cecal mass, which on laparotomy and resection turned out to be an appendiceal abscess (Groopman 2008).

The right renal mass apparently appeased the search satisfaction bias so that the appendiceal abnormality was not appreciated on the first CT scan.

Ashman Experiment – Search Satisfaction Bias

In 2000, Carol Ashman published a study demonstrating search satisfaction in skeletal radiology. Her subjects consisted of 10 radiology residents, 2 attending radiologists, and 13 orthopedic surgery residents. The subjects had 75 minutes to interpret 30 bone x-rays.

Of the 30 radiographs, 15 contained one significant diagnosis, 11 contained two significant diagnoses, and four radiographs contained three significant diagnoses. Most cases came from emergency department visits of patients presenting with pain.

The mean score for the radiographs with a single diagnosis was 11.25 of 15, with a standard deviation of 3.35. The mean score for the detection of at least one diagnosis on radiographs with two or three diagnoses was 11.72 of 15, with a standard deviation of 3.42. However, the mean score for the detection of two or three diagnoses in the radiographs with multiple abnormalities was only 6.12 of 15, with a standard deviation of 2.49.

Ashman's findings were
- The physician subjects showed a search satisfaction response for x-rays with two diagnoses, and the search satisfaction response increased for x-rays with three diagnoses.
- The false-positive rate increased with the time taken for search while the true-positive rate did not.

- Attending radiologists and upper level residents showed the search satisfaction effect to only a slightly lower degree than did lower level residents (Ashman 2000).

In brief, Ashman's findings supported the search satisfaction effect; and, the similarity of the effect between the *attending radiologists-upper level residents group* and the *lower level residents group* supported the effect's status as a true cognitive bias.

Countermeasures – Search Satisfaction Bias

The similarity in degree of the effect between the more and less experienced physicians in the Ashman study supports the status of the effect as a true cognitive bias, not just a consequence of carelessness or ignorance. This makes it difficult to address with primitive exhortations such as "Wake up and pay attention."

The simplest countermeasure to the search satisfaction bias is that once a target is found, **keep asking if there is something more** (Cognitive Bias 2014).

Probably more effective, given the status of the search satisfaction phenomenon as a true cognitive bias, is to adopt **checklists** or structured reporting (Pearson 2017; Kim 2014). A problem with checklists is the tendency to make them all-inclusive. Then, when the checklist is overwhelming, the tendency is to rush through and check boxes mechanically.

Structured reporting templates may be a better option to encourage active engagement of the reporter.
- Quattrocchi and his group retrospectively compared structured reporting with the usual free-text narrative for reporting extra-spinal incidental findings in lumbar spine MRIs. They utilized 3000 archived MRI reports and found 82% of E3 and 89% of E4 extra-spinal incidental findings unreported with the free-text narrative approach. (E3 findings are likely benign but indeterminate or incompletely characterized for which clinical correlation and further work-up *could* be indicated. E4 findings are potentially important findings *requiring* further work-up and communication to the referring physician) (Quattrocchi 2013).
- Semaan and his group performed a similar study using 3024 lumbar spine MRIs done for low back pain. They found, with non-structured reporting, an overall non-detection rate of 40% and an E4 non-detection rate of 38.6% (Semann 2015).

Another option is to **catalogue common oversights and design specific interventions** to reduce these (Pearson 2017; Kim 2014). In this case, checklists can be shortened to list only the common oversights, much the way surgical consent forms list only the common complications.

Interestingly, Fleck's experiments showed that increasing time pressure increases manifestations of search satisfaction bias. On the other hand, Ashman's study showed that increasing allotted time increased false-positive errors but did not increase true-positive findings. This conflict requires more investigation. Perhaps there is an **optimum examination time** for each particular radiographic or imaging study, an optimum up to which increasing time reduces search satisfaction and increases accuracy but beyond which it only increases false-positives. Certainly more studies of this phenomenon are required.

Conclusion

Search satisfaction bias is embodied in the admonition that the easiest fracture to miss is the second one. It is significant in medicine where physiological systems are interdependent and multiple problems can occur simultaneously. The search satisfaction bias has been described here and multiple countermeasures, from the simple to the sophisticated, have been discussed.

References

Cognitive bias. (2014, February 09). Retrieved July 03, 2017, from http://www.ganfyd.org/index.php?title=Cognitive_bias

Fleck, M. S., Samei, E., & Mitroff, S. R. (2010). Generalized "satisfaction of search": Adverse influences on dual-target search accuracy. Journal of Experimental Psychology: Applied,16(1), 60-71. doi:10.1037/a0018629

Groopman, J., & Hartzband, P. (2008, May). Beware of 'search satisfaction,' a common cognitive error. Retrieved July 3, 2017, from acpinternist.org/mindfulmedicine/bewareof search satisfaction
ACP Internist Mindful Medicine May 2008 Groopman, Hartzband

Gunderman, R. B. (2009). Biases in Radiologic Reasoning. American Journal of Roentgenology,192(3), 561-564. doi:10.2214/ajr.08.1220

Kim, Y. W., & Mansfield, L. T. (2014). Fool Me Twice: Delayed Diagnoses in Radiology With Emphasis on Perpetuated Errors. American Journal of Roentgenology,202(3), 465-470. doi:10.2214/ajr.13.11493

Pearson, D. (2017, January 30). 5 cognitive biases common to radiology-and how to beat them back. Retrieved July 03, 2017, from http://www.healthimaging.com/topics/diagnostic-imaging/5-cognitive-biases-common-radiology%E2%80%94and-how-counter-them

Quattrocchi, C. C., Giona, A., Martino, A. C., Errante, Y., Scarciolla, L., Mallio, C. A., . . . Zobel, B. B. (2013). Extra-spinal incidental findings at lumbar spine MRI in the general population: a large cohort study. *Insights into Imaging,4*(3), 301-308. doi:10.1007/s13244-013-0234-z

Semaan, H. B., Bieszczad, J. E., Obri, T., Aldinger, P. K., Bazerbashi, M. F., Al-Natour, M. S., & Elgafy, H. (2015). Incidental Extraspinal Findings at Lumbar Spine Magnetic Resonance Imaging. *Spine,40*(18), 1436-1443. doi:10.1097/brs.0000000000001024

Chapter 14: Representativeness Bias and Base-Rate Neglect

Representativeness Bias

Representativeness bias is a substitution heuristic. It i**s the substitution of similarity to a stereotype for probability of occurrence,** substitution of a simpler question for a more complex question. The simple question is **how similar something is to the stereotype of a class**. The more complex question is how probable something is to be a member of that class (Tversky and Kahneman 1974).

Common Example and Tom W Experiment – Representativeness Bias

Kahneman and Tversky's subjects were 114 graduate students in psychology from three US universities. They presented them with a **description of fictitious Tom W** whom they described as intelligent but lacking creativity, neat, given to corny puns, showing little empathy, not enjoying social interacting, and self-centered but moral. They indicated to the subjects that Tom W was currently a graduate student.

The researchers next presented the subjects with a list of 9 fields of study: business administration, computer science, engineering, humanities and education, law, library science, medicine, physical and life sciences, and social science and social work.

Kahneman and Tversky then asked the subjects to rank the above nine disciplines in the order of the *probability* with which Tom W was likely to be a student in that department of the university.

The subjects listed the mean order as computer science, engineering, physical and life sciences, business administration, library science, law, medicine, humanities and education, and social science and social work. Moreover, greater than 95% of the graduate student subjects judged that Tom W was more likely to be studying computer science than humanities, though they were certainly aware that there were many more graduate students in humanities and education.

Medical Example – Representativeness Bias

Stephen Novella makes the point that **myocardial infarctions in women** may be under diagnosed because women do not fit the stereotype of the typical MI patient.

Since 1984, the annual cardiovascular disease mortality rate has remained greater for women than men. One reason has been "under diagnosis" (Mehta 2016). Stephen Novella related this under diagnosis to the representativeness bias in that women do not fit the stereotype of the typical MI patient (Novella 2013). Fortunately, over recent years, the increased mortality rate has been abating; but this is more likely because the stereotype is changing than because the representativeness bias is subsiding.

Impact – Representativeness Bias

The major impact of the representativeness bias is that it bases *probability* on an irrelevant similarity to a stereotype rather than upon relevant base-rate information. In other words, it promotes base-rate neglect, our next topic.

Base-Rate Neglect

Base-rate neglect is the tendency, when presented with general information and specific information, **to under-weigh the general information and over-weigh the specific information**. It is, in a sense, missing the forest for the trees.

Common Example

A senior physician cited base-rate neglect in an incident recalled from early in the author's experience.

The physician, while working at the hospital, received a phone call that his **teen-aged son, who recently had a viral infection, was in the emergency room with chest pain**. A neophyte nurse on the phone told him not to worry because she did not think that the young man was having a myocardial infarct. The senior physician was taken aback by this comment and replied cynically, "In an 18 year-old with a recent viral infection and chest discomfort, you think of pericarditis, not myocardial infarct."

Linda Experiment – Base-Rate Neglect

In the **Linda Experiment** (Tversky and Kahneman 1983), the investigators presented to 88 undergraduates at the University of British Columbia this profile: Linda is 31 years old, single, outspoken, and very bright. She majored in philosophy. As a student, she was deeply concerned with issues of discrimination and social justice, and participated in anti-nuclear demonstrations.

The investigators then gave the undergraduates these eight statements about Linda:

- Linda is a teacher in elementary school.
- Linda works in a bookstore and takes yoga classes.
- Linda is active in the feminist movement.
- Linda is a psychiatric social worker.
- Linda is a member of the League of Women Voters.
- Linda is a bank teller.
- Linda is an insurance salesperson.
- Linda is a bank teller and is active in the feminist movement.

The researchers asked the undergraduates to rank the eight statements according to "the degree to which Linda resembles the typical member of that class." 85% of the undergraduates ranked "Linda is active in the feminist movement" higher than "**Linda is a bank teller and is active in the feminist movement,**" which they, in turn, **ranked higher than "Linda is a bank teller."**

However, the set of bank tellers who are feminists is clearly a subset of the set of bank tellers, so it is impossible to be more likely to be a feminist bank teller than it is to be just a bank teller. The undergraduates in this study exhibited base-rate neglect.

Engineer/Lawyer Experiment – Base-Rate Neglect

In the **engineer/lawyer experiment**, the same investigators (Tversky and Kahneman 1974) presented several individuals with brief personality descriptions of individuals allegedly sampled at random from a group of 100 professionals, all either engineers or lawyers. They asked the subjects to determine for each profile, whether the profile more probably belonged to an engineer or a lawyer.

One group of subjects was told that the 100 professionals consisted of 70 engineers and 30 lawyers. The other group was told that the 100 professionals consisted of 70 lawyers and 30 engineers. The subjects in the two groups made essentially the same probability judgments despite the fact that the compositions of the two groups were different. They ignored the base-rate information.

Medical Examples of Base-Rate Neglect

Anecdotal Examples

Dr. Theodore Woodward, professor at the University of Maryland School of Medicine in the late 1940s, counseled his interns against base rate neglect when he cautioned them, **"When you hear hoof beats, think of horses not zebras"** (Sotos 2006, p. 1). The point of Woodward's admonition was that although the equine's size is small or its gallop is slow for a horse, the fact remains that in Baltimore, Maryland, in the 1940s, the animal is still much more likely to be a horse than a zebra.

A subtler example of base-rate neglect is demonstrated by the **injudicious use of screening procedures**. Screening procedures are done on patients without symptoms. The intent of screening is to identify the presence of disease before symptoms develop and at a time sufficiently early to increase the likelihood of successful treatment.

The shortcoming in this seemingly prudent enterprise is that it neglects to quantify the base-rate and deleterious consequences of the disease being addressed. Neither does it specify the false positive rate and deleterious consequences of false positive test results. If the disease is rare in the population being tested, if some test false positives are inevitable, and if consequences of false positives are significant, then testing everyone may cause more damage than the disease itself. Moreover, testing may divert money and personnel that would be more productively spent treating the disease in question, and additional diseases as well.

In other words, if the screening is done on a population with a very small base-rate of a disease, there is a much greater probability of having a test response representative of the disease than the probability of having the disease itself.

Case Examples

These examples are selected from among those presented in *Avoiding Errors in General Practice* (Barraclough et al 2013, p. 113 and p 82 in Kindle edition). They illustrate unfortunate cases of base-rate neglect.

Elderly Woman with Fractured Hip

Case

May was 79 years old when she consulted Dr. Ali after tripping. Her left hip was painful with bruising over the left buttock and tenderness to palpation over the left hip. Even a week later, she had significant pain unrelieved by acetaminophen and ibuprofen. Three years previously, she had had a right total hip replacement. Dr. Ali evaluated her and prescribed acetaminophen with dihydrocodeine.

Ten days later, she had taken to her bed. This time Dr. Grant saw her. He diagnosed a urinary tract infection, prescribed trimethoprim for the urinary infection, and referred her to physical therapy for the hip. On her third visit to physical therapy, she stumbled on leaving the session and reported worsened pain.

X-ray revealed an impacted sub-capital fracture. May underwent left total hip replacement.

Commentary

Drs. Ali and Grant were seduced by base-rate neglect. Apparently, because they did not find leg length shortening on physical examination, they **overlooked the fact that the base-rate probability of fracture was very high for a 79 year-old female who had recently sustained trauma sufficient to cause bruising** and substantial pain. Leg length shortening might not be observed with an impacted sub-capital fracture; and, it certainly does not justify neglecting the fact that she falls into a class with a high base-rate probability for sustaining a fracture.

Middle-Aged Woman with Back Pain

Case

Angela had been experiencing increasing lumbar pain of 4 months duration when she consulted Dr. Ahmed. She had had breast cancer successfully treated 18 years previously.

Dr. Ahmed obtained blood tests and an x-ray of the lumbar spine. The lumbar spine film showed a bone cyst in the third lumbar vertebra and the radiologist's report suggested multiple myeloma blood screening. The multiple myeloma blood screening returned negative.

Three months later, Angela returned and saw Dr. Ahmed's colleague. She was in severe pain and had lost weight. She also had right leg weakness and difficulty passing urine.

Angela was admitted to hospital and determined to have vertebral metastasis at L3 and L4 with nerve root compression. She underwent emergency radiation therapy, but had residual urinary incontinence and right leg weakness.

Commentary

Dr. Ahmed's records contained Angela's history of breast cancer, but the background information submitted to the radiologist did not contain this information. Consequently, from radiographic appearance alone, the radiologist reported the x-ray to be consistent with multiple myeloma.

Nevertheless, Dr. Ahmed had the history of breast cancer but followed the radiologist's suggestion of myeloma screen. Certainly, this was an instance of availability bias.

Dr. Ahmed was then influenced by base-rate neglect. The probability of spine metastases in patients with a history of breast cancer is 4.06% for patients in their 40s and 50s and 6.88% for patients in their 60s and 70s (Aebi 2003). On the contrary, the probability of multiple myeloma in the same populations is only 0.003% (Shah 2016). **Breast cancer metastasis to the spine was over 1000 times more likely than multiple myeloma**.

Had it not been for base-rate neglect, Ahmed would have challenged the radiologists recommendation, verified that the radiologist had had the relevant facts before reading the x-ray, followed up with bone scan, and further pursued the metastatic disease work-up.

The real power of the base-rate is that it helps overcome vulnerability to the unknown unknowns. The supposition is that the unknown unknowns will be random and that they will, with a large number or over a significant period of time, cancel one another leaving the base rate as the principle influence. Consequently, Dr. Ahmed may not have been able to know that the radiologist did not have all the relevant information; but sticking close to the base-rate would have enabled him to deal appropriately with the situation.

Base-Rate Neglect Countermeasures

A significant countermeasure to base-rate neglect is **resisting the temptation to dismiss the information contained in the base-rate** with the statement that every case is unique (Kahneman 2015, p. 249 Kindle edition). This frequent argument discards substantial information. Certainly, everyone thinks that their marriage will be different or that their patient will respond differently, but the base-rate contains the information of all these individual instances.

Another significant countermeasure to base-rate neglect is the **demographic profile and history of the patient**. There seems a dangerous inclination to underrate history and demographics and rely on testing. Somehow, test results seem to be scientific (authority bias) while history seems to be simply social information. However, Angela's history of breast cancer, unavailable to the radiologist, made a difference. Angela's test results of "bone cyst" and negative blood markers for multiple myeloma did more harm than good because they were not guided by the base-rate.

The important advice given by Kahneman is that worthless information (how representative something is of its class) should be treated no differently from no information; and, **when there are doubts about the quality of the evidence, let judgments of probability stay close to the base-rate** (Kahneman 2015, p. 153).

Conclusion

Base-rate neglect is a bias that dismisses the substantial information contained in the base-rate. This information can be critical to making a diagnosis. Base-rate information is an effective tool in dealing with unknown unknowns. Information in the base-rate guides the appropriate selection of tests and thus provides protection from wrong conclusions suggested by misleading results of inappropriate tests.

References

Aebi, M. (2003). Spinal metastasis in the elderly. *European Spine Journal, 12*(0). doi:10.1007/s00586-003-0609-9

Barraclough, K. (2013). *Avoiding errors in general practice*. Chichester, West Sussex: Wiley-Blackwell.

Groopman, J. E. (2010). *How doctors think*. Carlton North, Vic.: Scribe Publications.

Kahneman, D., & Tversky, A. (july 1973). On the psychology of prediction. Psychological Reiew,80(4), 237-251. doi:10.1017/cbo9780511809477.005

Kahneman, D. (2015). *Thinking, fast and slow*. New York: Farrar, Straus and Giroux.

Mehta, L. S., Beckie, T. M., Devon, H. A., Grines, C. L., Krumholz, H. M., Johnson, M. N., . . . Wenger, N. K. (2016). Acute Myocardial Infarction in Women. Circulation,133(9), 916-947. doi:10.1161/cir.0000000000000351

Novella, S. (2013, March 20). Clinical Decision-Making Part III. Retrieved May 10, 2017, from https://sciencebasedmedicine.org/clinical-decision-making-part-iii/

Shah, Dhaval et al (2016) Multiple Myeloma Guidelines: Diagnosis, Treatment, Management of Multiple Myeloma–related Bone Disease. (2016, June 01). Retrieved April 02, 2017, from http://emedicine.medscape.com/article/2500014-overview

Sotos, J. G. (2006). *Zebra cards: an aid to obscure diagnosis*. Mt. Vernon, VA: Mt. Vernon Book Systems.

Tversky, A., & Kahneman, D. (1974). Judgment under Uncertainty: Heuristics and Biases. *Science, 185*(4157), 1124-1131. doi:10.1126/science.185.4157.1124

Tversky, A., & Kahneman, D. (1983). Extensional versus intuitive reasoning: The conjunction fallacy in probability judgment. *Psychological Review, 90*(4), 293-315. doi:10.1037//0033-295x.90.4.293

Further Reading

Barraclough, K. (2013). *Avoiding errors in general practice*. Chichester, West Sussex: Wiley-Blackwell.

Groopman, J. E. (2010). *How doctors think*. Carlton North, Vic.: Scribe Publications.

Kahneman, D. (2015). *Thinking, fast and slow*. New York: Farrar, Straus and Giroux.

Tversky, A., & Kahneman, D. (1974). Judgment under Uncertainty: Heuristics and Biases. *Science, 185*(4157), 1124-1131. doi:10.1126/science.185.4157.1124

Logical Fallacies

Chapter 15: Logical Fallacies – Affirming the Consequent, Post Hoc Fallacy, and Toupee Fallacy

Logical Fallacies

While the last several chapters have addressed psychological biases, these three chapters address logical fallacies.

Whereas **psychological biases are concerned with errors of information acquisition, logical fallacies are concerned with errors of information manipulation**. While psychological biases lead to the acquisition of false information, logical fallacies can produce false conclusions from true information. Biases lead to false premises; fallacies lead to false conclusions from true premises.

Finally since psychological biases occur at the very basic and less attentional level of information acquisition, countermeasures addressed to attention, such as the exhortation "Be more careful," are poorly effective. By contrast, **since logical fallacies occur at the higher, more attentional level of information manipulation, education about fallacy mechanics and intensification of attention are far more effective as countermeasures**. Consequently, these three chapters examine the mechanics of logical fallacies and promote attention to them.

Logical fallacies were first categorized by Aristotle (384 BCE – 322 BCE) in *On Sophistical Refutations*, a text in his *Organon*. There he lists about a dozen logical fallacies. We still fall into these fallacies almost 2400 years later.

Affirming the Consequent Fallacy

In an "if ... then" statement, the element following the "if" is called the *antecedent* and the element following the "then" is called the *consequent*. Thus, consider the statement, "If a municipality is a city in Illinois, then it is a city in the US." Here the element "If a municipality is a city in Illinois" is the antecedent while the element "it is a city in the US" is the consequent. Again, consider the statement "If two triangles have three equal sides, then they have equal areas." Here, the element "two triangles have three equal sides" is the antecedent, while the element "they have equal areas" is the consequent.

Affirming the *antecedent* always leads to a valid argument. Thus, when the "if ... then" statement is true and the antecedent is true, the consequent must be true.

Consequently, since any city in Illinois is a city in the US, and Chicago is a city in Illinois, then Chicago is a city in the US. Similarly, Sam's 3 cm – 4 cm – 5 cm triangle and Sally's 3 cm – 4 cm – 5 cm triangle, since they have three equal sides, have equal areas.

Further, negating the consequent always leads to a valid argument. Thus, since Mumbai is not a city in the US, it is not a city in Illinois. Again, if Sam's triangle and Sally's triangle do not have equal areas, then they do not have equal sides.

However, while affirming the *antecedent* and *negating the* consequent are both valid reasoning steps, **affirming the *consequent* is a logical fallacy**. Because Seattle is a city in the US does not imply that it is a city in Illinois. Again, two triangles having equal areas do not necessarily have corresponding equal sides.

Common Example of Affirming the Consequent

A common example of affirming the consequent would be taking the *converse* of the triangle statement, namely, that if two triangles have equal areas, they have three equal sides. Thus, suppose that Seth draws *any* triangle and that Sarah draws an *equilateral* triangle of equal area (geometric methods make possible the construction of an equilateral triangle with area equal to any given triangle). However, Sarah's triangle is equilateral while Seth's is not, so the two triangles do not have three corresponding equal sides. This is the logical fallacy.

Medical Example of Affirming the Consequent

Many medical examples of affirming the consequent involve rash diagnosis.

Streptococcal pharyngitis manifests as sore throat. "This patient has a sore throat, so he has streptococcal pharyngitis." This is possibly true, but the sore throat may be viral or may be from dry indoor wintertime air.

This is the reason for a rapid strep test, which, if positive, will surely diagnose streptococcal pharyngitis. Oops, affirming the consequent again! The positive rapid strep test may indicate only that the patient is a strep carrier.

In interpreting EKGs, EEGs, chest x-rays, and other studies, cardiologists, neurologists, and radiologists typically avoid affirming the consequent by reporting that the study they are interpreting is "consistent with" rather than indicative of a given diagnosis.

Negating the Antecedent Fallacy

While, as previously mentioned, **negating the consequent *is* valid deduction; nevertheless, negating the antecedent *is not* valid. One cannot say that since any city in Illinois is a city in the US, and Milwaukee is not a city in Illinois, then Milwaukee is not a city in the US**. Similarly, one cannot say that since Sam's 1 cm – 12 cm – 12.05 cm right triangle and Sally's 3 cm – 4 cm – 5 cm triangle do *not* have three equal sides, they do *not* have equal areas.

Negating the antecedent is *not* grounds for negating the consequent. The antecedent is evidence that supports the conclusion. Carl Sagan referenced the argument that UFOs must exist since there is no compelling evidence that they do not. He regarded this conclusion as impatience with ambiguity and, with respect to it, he famously quipped, **"Absence of evidence is not evidence of absence"** (Sagan 1997, p 200).

Appeal to Ignorance

Negating the antecedent is related in classical logic to **appeal to ignorance**. Often this involves **proposing vague, confusing, or meaningless "evidence"** and arguing that some bizarre conclusion is justified. Sometimes this involves proposing untestable propositions as evidence and claiming that this justifies some conclusion.

Medical examples of argument from ignorance unfortunately occur. When AIDS was new, rampant, and poorly understood in the 1980s, some argued that the disease was God's wrath against the gay community. Other untestable explanations are the **phlogiston explanation of fire**, the caloric explanation of heat, and the miasma explanation of disease.

The fact remains that the burden of proof lies on the proposer of the argument to demonstrate its truth and that an explanation must be *disprovable*.

Post Hoc Fallacy

The *Post Hoc* fallacy receives its name from the Latin *Post Hoc Ergo Propter Hoc*, **"after this therefore on account of this."** It imputes causality to time sequence. It claims that when an event occurs, the immediately preceding event must be the cause.

The *post* hoc fallacy is a subcase of affirming the consequent. Its form is "If A causes B, then A precedes B. But A preceded B, therefore A caused B."

Common Examples of *Post Hoc* Fallacy

Soon after **Johnny Cochran**, famous defense attorney in the OJ Simpson Case, **died of a malignant brain tumor, there was a renaissance of the belief that cell phones cause brain cancer**. After all, was not Cochran frequently seen speaking on the cell phone? Certainly, but was not he also frequently seen walking quickly, talking to OJ, and carrying a leather briefcase?

Sandy Macaskill chronicled some of the most interesting soccer superstitions. He recounts the story of **Brazilian soccer star Pelé who fell into a slump after giving one of his shirts to a fan.** Convinced that this gift caused his slump, Pelé sent a friend to recover the shirt. After the friend returned Pelé's shirt to him, Pelé's slump ended. But, in reality, the friend had been unable to recover the shirt and returned to Pelé one of Pelé's old shirts instead (Macaskill 2009).

Medical Example of *Post Hoc* Fallacy

Kim and Gallis 1989 have studied fallacies they have seen in **infectious disease** practice. Here is one relevant to the *post hoc* fallacy and affirming the consequent.

A 35 year-old woman was admitted to hospital with headache, dizziness, and bilateral facial palsies. Two months earlier, she had left Bell's palsy partially responsive to prednisone. Neurological examination revealed predominately right-sided cranial nerve VII palsy. CT and MRI of the head were normal. Cerebrospinal fluid (CSF) examination revealed elevated protein and white blood cell (WBC) count of $10/mm^3$. CSF cultures were negative for bacteria, fungi, and mycobacteria, while VDRL and cytologies were negative. Chest x-ray showed hilar adenopathy without parenchymal disease and tuberculin skin test was negative.

Although Lyme meningitis was considered unlikely, high dose penicillin (12-20 million units per day) was instituted. The patient showed resolution of headache and gradual improvement of her facial nerve palsies. Despite this "successful" trial, bronchoscopy was done and showed non-caseating granulomata. Penicillin was halted and prednisone was initiated for sarcoidosis of the central nervous system (Kim and Gallis 1989).

Instead of "*post hoc* fallacy" or "affirming the consequent," **Kim and Gallis refer to the fallacy as "response implies diagnosis."** Regardless of terminology, **this fallacy cautions against too much confidence in "trials of therapy".**

Toupee Fallacy

The toupee fallacy results when a conclusion is drawn from only part of the data under the supposition that this part of the data represents all of the data. The name derives from the most famous example of the fallacy: **"I can always tell a man with a toupee."** It is a fallacy because the **claimant does not know how many of deceptive toupees have escaped his identification**.

Common and Medical Examples of the Toupee Fallacy

Common examples of the toupee fallacy include such statements as
- I can always tell when you are lying.
- I can always spot a New Yorker.
- I can always tell when someone has been smoking.
- I can always identify the toupee fallacy.

Medical examples of the toupee fallacy include such statements as
- I can always tell when someone has had plastic surgery.
- I can always spot a malingerer.
- **I can always spot a drug-seeking patient.**

Examining the Toupee Fallacy

The toupee fallacy has been related to the confirmation bias (Novella 2012, p. 73). It has also been related to rash generalization and conclusion from inadequate statistical sample.

We find an additional relationship, namely, to the fallacy of affirming the consequent. The reasoning is as follows: "Every time I have judged a man to be wearing a toupee, he has been, in fact, wearing one. Therefore, if a man is wearing a toupee, I will detect it." This is certainly an instance of affirming the consequent.

Falling victim to the toupee fallacy involves **confusing a sufficient condition with a necessary condition**. Suppose an observer has a perfect positive record, that is, every time the observer has judged a subject to be wearing a toupee, then the subject was, in fact, wearing one. Here the observer's judgment is a **sufficient condition** for the conclusion that the subject is wearing a toupee.

However, the observer's judgment is not a **necessary condition**. A subject could be wearing a very convincing toupee without the observer recognizing it.

Another way of looking at this is to say that the perfect positive observer is **specific** in that the observer's positive identification is never wrong. However, the observer is not **sensitive** in that some toupee instances escape the observer's identification (Chapter 20 for more on sensitivity and specificity).

References

Kim, J. H., & Gallis, H. A. (1989). Observations on spiraling empiricism: Its causes, allure, and perils, with particular reference to antibiotic therapy. The American Journal of Medicine,87, 201-206. doi:10.1016/0002-9343(89)90572-x

Macaskill, S. (2009, February 25). Top 10: Football superstitions to rival Arsenal's Kolo Toure. The Telegraph.

Novella, S. (2012). Your deceptive mind: a scientific guide to critical thinking skills. Chantilly, VA: Teaching Company.

Sagan, C. (1997). The demon-haunted world. New York: Random House.

Further Reading

Novella, S. (2012). Your deceptive mind: a scientific guide to critical thinking skills. Chantilly, VA: Teaching Company.

Chapter 16: Logical Fallacies – "Straw Man" and Begging the Question

"Straw Man" Fallacy

The **"Straw Man" fallacy is a logical error in which a strong argument is sidestepped and a weaker or ludicrous version of that argument is substituted and addressed**.

Common Examples of "Straw Man" Fallacy

Examples of the "Straw Man" fallacy are rife in daily life. **Arguments that guns should be more closely regulated, are met with the response "Then only criminals will have guns."** Here, the premise that all guns should be illegal is substituted for the premise that guns should be more closely regulated.

Bishop Samuel Wilberforce, in 1860, during a debate on evolution with Thomas Henry Huxley, **asked Huxley whether it was on his grandfather's or his grandmother's side that Huxley was descended from an ape**. Here the premise that evolution occurred in historical time is substituted for the premise that evolution predated historical time. Additionally, the premise of direct descent is substituted for the premise of descent from a single common ancestor.

Sometimes the substituted premise is only implied. Coca-Cola was made with coca leaf extract since 1886 but the process to remove all cocaine from coca leaf extract was not perfected until 1929. Therefore, it seems that Coca-Cola contained cocaine during its early years. Nevertheless, the Coca-Cola Company denies that the beverage ever contained cocaine (Palermo 2013). This is reconcilable only if the company is arguing that the beverage never contained *added* cocaine. However, this is a substitution for the original premise.

It is evident from the above examples that the "Straw Man" fallacy may be involved any time there is a seeming pretense to misunderstand the question.

Medical Examples of "Straw Man" Fallacy

In the Coca-Cola example, the substituted premise was implied. However, in the following medical example, the primary premise, the one being substituted for, is implied.

Prilosec[TM] (omeprazole) is a proton pump inhibitor, a medication to reduce acid secretion in the stomach. It consists of two isomers, left-handed and right-handed versions of the same molecule. The left-handed molecule is a stronger proton pump inhibitor than the right-handed molecule.

Nexium[TM] (esomeprazole) is just the isolated more potent left-handed version of the molecule that was introduced at a substantially higher price when Prilosec went off patent. Prilosec is now sold over the counter.

Surprisingly, AstraZenica, manufacturer of both Nexium and omeprazole (Prilosec), conducted head-to-head trials between the two drugs and announced that **erosive esophagitis healed in 94% of patients on Nexium vs. 84% on omeprazole**, again in 94% of patients on Nexium vs. 87% on omeprazole, and 92% of patients on Nexium vs. 90% on omeprazole (Nexium Delivers Proven Healing 2017).

Nevertheless, review of the studies shows that AstraZenica in each case compared 40 mg of Nexium with 20 mg of omeprazole. Recall, however, that Nexium (esomeprazole) is the more potent component of omeprazole, so an equal dose alone should have been more effective, without need of a double-dose, which still only showed marginal advantage.

In conclusion, the primary question here was "Is Nexium a more effective gastric acid suppressor than omeprazole (in equal doses)? The published report substitutes the question "Is Nexium a more effective gastric acid suppressor at double the dose?" It answers the question "Yes, it is [marginally]."

"Begging the Question" Fallacy

Begging the question is the fallacy of assuming the premise intended to be proved. The term is frequently misused. To beg a question is to commit a logical fallacy; it is *not* another way of saying to pose a question or to ask a question.

Common Examples of "Begging the Question" Fallacy

Possibly the most famous example of begging the question comes from Molière where his character in the comedy *Le Malade Imaginere* explains that **opium causes sleep because it has soporific properties** (Molière 1673)

One of the most trivial examples of begging the question is the supposed, but not seriously used, argument "God exists because the Bible says so."

However, the examples become subtler. Consider, "All abortion should be illegal because it kills a human being," which assumes that all fetuses are human beings.

More subtle still is the question begging epithet such as in the example "All abortion should be illegal because it kills an unborn child," which assumes that all fetuses are children. The epithet is a more subtle invocation of begging the question because when question begging is phrased as an argument, as in the Bible example, it invites challenge. When it is phrased as an epithet, it is built into a name, which, unless terribly offensive, is less likely to be challenged.

Medical Examples of "Begging the Question" Fallacy

Some medical examples of question begging involve citing symptoms as diagnoses. One such example would be **"His sore throat is due to pharyngitis."** This may escape notice since it resembles the valid diagnosis "His sore throat is due to streptococcal pharyngitis."

Medicine also has its share of question begging epithets. An example is the accusation "Joseph Smith, MD is a provider whose treatment is impersonal." Here, the idea of impersonal treatment is contained within the word "provider" that assumes he is a retailer or agent of services rather than a physician committed to patients.

A similar epithet-employing accusation is **"Mary Jones, MD must be negligent because she carries malpractice insurance."** Here the idea of negligence is contained within the word "malpractice," whereas it would have been absent from the less judgmental term "professional liability insurance."

A final example of the question-begging epithet is the term "benefits" used by some health insurance companies in the phrase "benefits provided." The question to be answered is are the services mentioned truly beneficial or just contractual services in exchange for money, services possibly insufficient or overpriced.

References

Molière (Writer). (1673). Le Malade Imaginere.
(1673), Act III, sc. iii.

Nexium Delivers Proven Healing of EE. (n.d.). Retrieved June 16, 2017, from https://www.nexiumtouchpoints.com/content/us/nexium/web/www-nexiumtouchpoints-com/en/nexium-information/healing-erosive-esophagitis

Palermo, E. (2013, December 16). Does Coca-Cola Contain Cocaine? Retrieved June 16, 2017, from https://www.livescience.com/41975-does-coca-cola-contain-cocaine.html

Chapter 17: Logical Fallacies – Faulty Analogy and Nirvana Fallacy

Faulty Analogy Fallacy

Faulty analogy is one of the most common logical fallacies. It **consists in drawing false conclusions by making inappropriate comparisons**. Faulty analogy assumes that because two things are alike in some respects, that they are also alike in other respects.

In 1860 Bishop Samuel Wilberforce and Thomas Henry Huxley debated evolution at the Oxford University Museum, In the debate, Wilberforce famously asked Huxley whether it from his grandmother's or grandfather's side that he claimed descent from a monkey. Wilberforce mistakenly compared Darwinian evolution of species through natural selection to human genealogy.

Analogies with True Conclusions

Some analogies yield true conclusions.

Geometry yields such an example. Among all rectangles with a fixed perimeter, the square has the maximum area. From this it might be analogically argued that among all six-sided solid structures with a fixed surface area, the cube has the maximum volume (Bartha 2013). Here the conclusion is true.

Astronomy yields another example of an analogy with a true conclusion. Although Copernicus's heliocentric theory was published 21 years before Galileo's birth, astronomers of Galileo's time still doubted Copernicus's conclusions. **Galileo**, however, supported Copernicus because he had observed in his telescope four moons orbiting Jupiter. He **argued that, analogous to the four moons orbiting Jupiter, the earth orbited the sun**.

Medicine yields another example of a true conclusion from an analogous argument. In 1934, Schaumann noted that morphine and meperidine had a similar molecular structure. He noted also that both seemed to induce upon mice an S-shaped tail curvature. **Schaumann inferred**, analogically and correctly, **that meperidine might have analgesic properties similar to morphine** (Bartha 2013) (Lembeck 1989) (Reynolds 1975).

Analogies with False Conclusions

Other analogies yield false conclusions.

Several common examples come to mind.
- "Meat is murder."
- Banning handguns makes as much sense as banning automobiles.
- "Pooches are children with fur."
- **Taking Holy Communion is cannibalism**.

Physics yields a famous example.
- **Just as water waves and sound waves are disturbances in a medium, light waves are disturbances in a medium**. This analogy persisted until Michelson and Morley's interferometer experiment offered contradictory evidence in 1887.

More examples emerge from armchair psychology.
- Observers of young lovers sometimes comment that opposites attract. However, this is a hasty analogy between inter-personality dynamics and electrostatic physics.
- Observers of children playing violent video games sometimes comment favorably, saying "It's better that they let off steam here." However, this is a hasty analogy between aggression in psychology and steam in fluid static physics.

Medicine has its own share of analogous arguments yielding false conclusions.
- For many years, children were believed to be simply miniature adults.
- **Hippocrates and centuries of successors believed the body to harbor four humors analogous to the four elements of earth, air, fire, and water.**
- A popular superstition, never scientifically accepted, discourages cancer surgery on the assumption that once air contacts a malignant tumor, it spreads like wildfire. A fresh air supply hastens the spread of a blaze, not of a tumor. This is a hasty analogy between oncologic surgery and fire science.

Is There a Logic of Analogies?

A logic of analogies would be of great benefit. At the least, it would enable us to separate analogies rendering true conclusions from analogies rendering untrue conclusions. In other words, at the least, it would be a *logic of critique*. At the most, it would enable us to input true statements into a reliable computational engine and always output true conclusions. In other words, at the most, it would be a *logic of discovery*.

History is replete with efforts to develop a logic of analogies. Philosophers, psychologists, mathematicians, and computer scientists have all addressed the problem. It has even been a topic in artificial intelligence research.

Aristotle considered the problem in the fourth century BC in *Rhetoric, Prior Analytics,* and *Topics* (Bartha 2013)(Aristotle and Barnes 1985). Thereafter, David Hume addressed the problem in the eighteenth century in *Dialogues Concerning Natural Religion* (Hume 1779). John Stuart Mill considered the problem mid-nineteenth century in *A System of Logic* (Mill 1875). Finally, British mathematician and philosopher Mary Hesse, in the mid-twentieth century created a large body of work on the subject (Hesse 1966).

Nevertheless, to date **no one has been able to formulate an acceptable rule or set of rules for valid analogical inferences** (Bartha 2013).

Conclusion on Analogy Fallacy

It is unfortunate that the term "faulty analogy" has established itself so firmly in usage. The term suggests that a criterion has been formulated to distinguish faulty analogy from valid analogy. However, no such objective criterion, or logic of analogies, has ever been established.

In the absence of an objective criterion, arbitrary and subjective results cannot be excluded. Further, the confirmation bias would favor analogies resulting in desired conclusions being regarded as valid and analogies resulting in undesired conclusions being regarded as "faulty." Consequently, unless and until such a criterion is constructed, **analogical inferences should not be trusted**.

Nirvana Fallacy

Another frequent fallacy is the Nirvana Fallacy. The **Nirvana fallacy compares a practical *good* solution to an impractical or hypothetical *perfect* solution. It then argues that the imperfect solution is not worth pursuing**. The Nirvana fallacy often appears in a context in which there is reluctance to take reasonable precautions. The fallacy is also known as the "Perfect Solution Fallacy."

Voltaire is widely credited with the saying "the better is the enemy of the good" in *Dictionnaire philosophique* (Philosophical Dictionary) 1770. However, the phrase appears earlier in Shakespeare's *King Lear* 1605 and earlier still in Orlando Pescetti's *Proverbi italiani* (Italian Proverbs) 1603.

Nirvana Fallacy – Narrow Examples

The Nirvana fallacy exhibits itself in both narrow and broad examples. In the narrow case, the fallacy compares an imperfect, but practical and good, solution against a perfect, but impractical or hypothetical, solution *to the same problem*.

An initial example is "I'm not stopping smoking. People like Andy Kaufman didn't smoke and died of lung cancer anyway." Another example is **"I'm not locking my doors at night. You could lock your doors and get robbed anyway."** Similar examples include wearing seat belts while driving and getting a flu shot.

A last example is "Making guns difficult to obtain is useless as a criminal could get a gun anyway."

Nirvana Fallacy – Broad Example

In the broad case, the fallacy compares an imperfect, but practical and good, solution against a perfect, but impractical or hypothetical, solution *to any problem*.

Recently, after a national spate of mass killings involving automatic weapons followed by a local irresponsible sale of two such weapons, a letter to the editor appeared in the city newspaper criticizing the easy availability of automatic weapons.

The author identified himself as a physician as he quoted similar positions published as an editorial in the *Journal of the American Medical Association Internal Medicine* and as a policy statement of the American Academy of Pediatrics. There followed in the paper angry responses stating that **easy availability of automatic weapons should not be questioned since an equivalent number of deaths nationally were due to automobile accidents and medical accidents!**

Conclusion on Nirvana Fallacy

It seems that employing the Nirvana fallacy is a rationalization for a decision made on non-rational grounds. It is difficult to imagine that any American male would rationally choose smoking over not smoking after reading that not smoking reduces the risk in American males of lung cancer by 95.65% but not by 100% (following Lung Cancer Fact Sheet 2018). Certainly, **if the probability of winning an even money bet were 95.65%, no one would decline the bet because the probability was not 100%.**

Countermeasures and Conclusion - Logical Fallacies

Logical fallacies are unlike psychological biases. Logical fallacies deal with the manipulation of information and with the drawing of conclusions from information. Psychological biases deal with information acquisition. Logical fallacies occur more at the level of attention. Psychological biases occur more below the level of attention and so are more insidious.

Because of this, countermeasures to bias depend more on restructuring circumstances rather than intensifying attention. However, **countermeasures to fallacies consist of examining the mechanics of the fallacy and intensifying attention**. This has been the object of the last three chapters.

References Analogy Fallacy

Aristotle, & Barnes, J. (1985). *The complete works of Aristotle*. Princeton N.J.: Princeton University Press.

Bartha, P. (2013, June 25). Stanford Encyclopedia of Philosophy: Analogy and Analogical Reasoning. Retrieved December 29, 2017, from https://plato.stanford.edu/entries/reasoning-analogy/

Hesse, M. B. (1966). *Models and analogies in science*. Notre Dame (Ind.): University of Notre Dame Press.

Hume, D. (1779). *Dialogues concerning natural religion, by David Hume, ... The 2d edition*. London.

Lembeck, F. (1989). *Scientific alternatives to animal experiments*. Chichester: Ellis Horwood.
Mill, J. S. (1875). *A System of Logic ... Second edition*. London.

Lung Cancer Fact Sheet. (2018). Retrieved January 05, 2018, from http://www.lung.org/lung-health-and-diseases/lung-disease-lookup/lung-cancer/resource-library/lung-cancer-fact-sheet.html

Reynolds, A. K., & Randall, L. O. (1975). *Morphine and Related Drugs*. Toronto: University of Toronto Press.

Innumeracy

Chapter 18: Randomness, Uniformity, and the Sharpshooter Fallacy

Randomness and Uniformity

Randomness and uniformity are easily confused. The irregularities of small populations fade into invisibility in larger populations. Nevertheless, this is quickly forgotten and replaced by the assumption that the relative uniformity of large populations is reflected at every component level. The expectation of uniformity quickly extinguishes the ability to produce randomness and the ability to recognize randomness.

Difficulty Producing Randomness

Initially, **one might think that producing randomness is a simple task for the human brain. However, investigations show otherwise**.

Boland-Hutchinson Experiment

In 2000, Boland and Hutchinson published an experiment in which they asked university students with some statistical knowledge to generate randomly 25 digits from the set {0, 1, 2, 3, 4, 5, 6, 7, 8, 9}. The results were not random. The digit 0 had a less favored status than the other 9 digits. On the other hand, 1, 2, and 3 were surprisingly popular. Additionally, 70% of students failed to give the same digit twice in succession when in a random sample one would expect this to happen in 8% of cases.

Finally, the selections of each student were less variable than randomness would expect. There was a nonrandom tendency to balance the selections around the median. Specifically, 49% of the students balanced 12 or 13 digits less than the median when randomness would expect only 31% (Boland 2000).

Figurska Experiment

In 2008, Figurska and colleagues published an experiment in which 37 adult subjects were asked to dictate random digits from the set {0, 1, 2, 3, 4, 5, 6, 7, 8, 9}. A subject could continue so long as they liked, to a time limit of 10 minutes. If a subject ended before 10 minutes, their digits were recorded and they were asked to begin again until their total time reached 10 minutes.

Findings were that the mean frequency of any digit approached the frequency found in a computer-generated random number distribution. However, an analysis of pairs of neighboring digits, a and b in a sequence, revealed the following frequencies

- a = b occurred 7.6% whereas 10% would be expected randomly.
- a = b + 1 occurred 15.4% whereas 9% would be expected randomly.
- a = b - 1 occurred 16.9% whereas 9% would be expected randomly.

The investigators concluded that none of the results obtained by human subjects were truly random (Figurska 2008).

Difficulty Recognizing Randomness

Recognition of randomness would seem to be a relatively easy task. However, the reality is otherwise.

Purcell's Dots

Consider these images (Fig. 18.1) generated by Ed Purcell and appearing in Stephen Jay Gould's *Bully for Brontosaurus*. See if you can determine which is random.

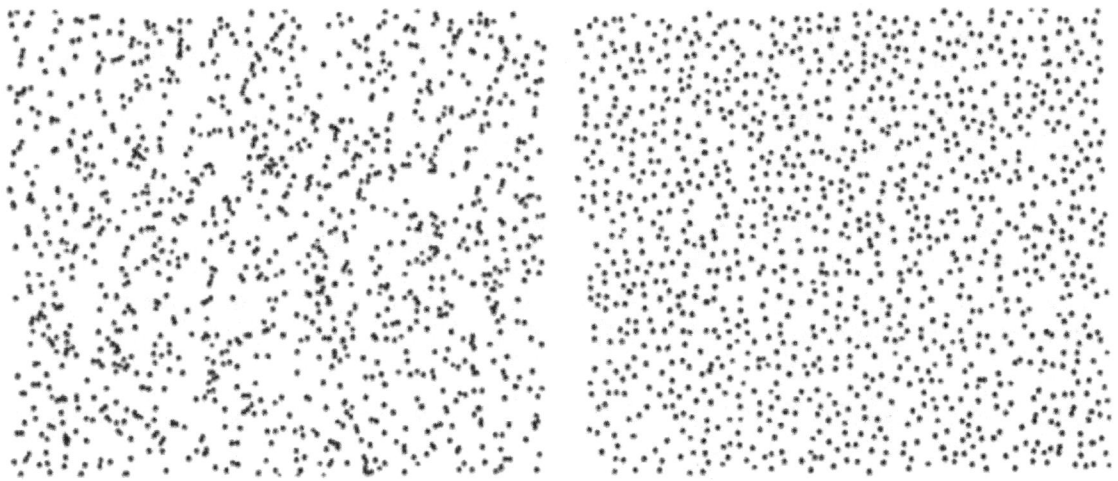

Fig. 18.1. From Stephen Jay Gould, 2001, *Bully for Brontosaurus*, p 266-267).

Have you decided?

Many people observe the clumps and filaments in the left image vs. the uniformity in the right image; they judge the left image to be organized and the right image to be random. However, this is a confusion of uniformity for randomness.

The left image is a representation of stars in the night sky and is random. The right image is a representation of glowworms on the ceiling of Waitomo Cave on the north island of New Zealand; it tends to uniformity as the organisms incline to equalize the distances between one another.

The images above are an example **that it is not unusual to perceive patterns in randomness**.

Wagenaar Experiment

In 1970, Willem Wagenaar published a study on the perception of randomness. He presented subjects with a large number of slides, each of which contained seven series of white and black dots on a grey background. For each of the slides the subjects were asked to respond which of the seven looked most random.

On each slide, one series had a 0.2 probability of two successive black dots or two successive white dots, one series had a 0.3 probability, one a 0.4 probability, and so on up to 0.8. In a random series, the probability is 0.5, just as the probability with a fair coin of flipping a head after a previous head is 0.5. Instead, the subjects judged the series with probability of 0.4 as being the most random (Wagenaar 1970).

The experiment demonstrated that the subjects saw randomness in patterns and patterns in randomness.

Feller Study

From June through October 1944, 2419 German V1 jet-propelled buzz bombs, launched from France and the Netherlands, fell on London. Maps of impact sites revealed clumps and gaps. British intelligence saw a pattern in this and was concerned that certain sites were avoided because they harbored German spies (Bhatia 2012).

Croatian-American mathematician William (Vilibald) Feller approached the problem and was able to determine that the pattern of London impacts was typical of a random process (Kahneman 2015, pp. 115-116).

The British Intelligence Service had perceived nonexistent patterns in randomness.

Gilovich Study

Basketball players, their fans, and their coaches tend to believe that streaks are the effect of a phenomenon known as the "hot hand." In 1985, Thomas Gilovich conducted a study to determine if this belief is justified.

To exemplify frequency of the "hot hand" belief, Gilovich and colleagues surveyed a total of 100 basketball-playing students from Cornell and Stanford universities. They found of the students that

- 91% believed a player has "a better chance of making a shot after having just made his last two or three shots than he does after having just missed his last two or three shots."
- 68% expressed essentially the same belief for free throws,
- 84% believed "it is important to pass the ball to someone who has just made several (two, three, or four) shots in a row."

Next, to determine if belief in the "hot hand" phenomenon is justified, Gilovich and colleagues examined data from the Philadelphia 76ers' season of 1980-1981. The investigators found that

- Following a hit, the probability of a hit at the next opportunity was 51%.
- Following a miss, the probability of a hit at the next opportunity was 54%.
- Following a "hot " period of three or four hits in the last four shots, the probability of a hit at the next opportunity was 50%.
- Following a "cold" period of three or four misses in the last four shots, the probability of a hit at the next opportunity was 57%.

Finally, the investigators became concerned that recent successes or failures might change the players' propensity to take only easy shots or to take increasingly more difficult shots. Investigators also felt that recent successes or failures might change the defensive measures against the players. To eliminate these influences, they studied only free throws of the Boston Celtics in the 1980-1981 and 1981-1982 seasons.

The free throw study on the Celtics showed no correlations "significantly different from zero" and provided "no evidence that the outcome of the second free throw is influenced by the outcome of the first free throw" (Gilovich 1985).

Basketball player, fans, and coaches, like Wagenaar's subjects and the British Intelligence Service, perceived patterns in randomness.

Difficulty Recognizing Randomness – Medical Examples

It is improbable for a coincidence to occur in a *given place* but not improbable for a coincidence to occur *someplace*.

It is improbable, in flipping a fair coin, to flip three successive heads in the next three flips (1 in 8), but not improbable to flip three successive heads in the next 24 flips (1 in 1). It is an error to retrospectively select the three consecutive heads, ignore the other flips, and conclude that the coin is not fair. **Error lies in identifying unusual incidents *in retrospect* and hypothesizing causal**

agency for them without ascertaining their true probability or corroborating a cause.

Cancer Clusters

True probability is easier to ascertain in coin flips than in epidemiological situations. In epidemiology, sometimes the best that can be expected is to identify a cluster, investigate it, and find a cause. When a cause cannot be found, random clustering remains a major consideration.

In 1854, John Snow saw a cluster of cholera cases in the Soho district of London in proximity to a water pump on Broad Street. Snow became suspicious, investigated further, and confirmed his suspicions about the pump. He alerted authorities, who disabled the pump, whereupon the cholera epidemic subsided.

In 1976, 24 people died and 130 sickened shortly after returning from an American Legion Convention at the Bellevue-Stratford Hotel in Philadelphia. The victims could have been lost among the 2000 conventioneers from all areas of the country. However, Dr. Ernest Campbell of Bloomsburg, Pennsylvania noted that three of his patients were among those sickened at the convention. He notified public health authorities, who identified *Legionella pneumophila* in the Bellevue-Stratford's air conditioning system.

However, clear-cut cases such as these have not been common in the investigations of cancer clusters. The discovery of clear cell carcinoma of the vagina or cervix of women whose mothers took diethylstilbestrol (DES) during pregnancy is a rare exception. Another exception is the discovery of mesothelioma in shipyard workers. Nevertheless, cases such as these have been highly unusual and the overwhelming majority of *perceived* clusters eventuate as false perceptions or as incapable of substantiation.

A 1990 study by Bender reviewed 400 possible clusters reported to the Minnesota Department of Health over the period 1981-1988. Of these, only 1% merited a full-scale epidemiologic study (Bender 1990).

In a study published in 1990, Caldwell noted that from 1961 until the study, the Centers for Disease Control investigated 108 cancer clusters from 29 states and five foreign countries. Nevertheless, CDC found no clear cause for any of the clusters (Caldwell 1990).

The American Cancer Society reports that **random patterns with no identified cause are the most common reason for a cancer cluster** (Cancer Clusters 2017).

Certainly, there are many cases in which cancer clusters are simply a consequence of randomness being different from uniformity.

Sharpshooter Fallacy

The **sharpshooter fallacy** gets its name from the conjured image of a man haphazardly shooting at the side of a barn. After producing a random array of bullet holes on the barn side, he strides up to the barn, selects one of the bullet holes (or, better, an area where a few bullet holes are clustered), draws a bull's eye around this, and proclaims that the bull's eye attests to the accuracy of his shooting.

This is obviously a case of imposing meaning upon nothing or upon the non-uniformity of randomness.

Goldacre's Medical Example

Ben Goldacre describes the unfortunate case of **Dutch pediatric nurse Lucia de Berk**. Ms. de Berk **spent six years in prison on seven counts of murder and three of attempted murder, convicted on only weak circumstantial evidence** (Goldacre 2011).

After finding seven deaths on her shifts in one hospital, prosecutors rushed to judgment, ignoring statistical information. In the three years before Lucia worked on the ward, there were seven deaths. In the three years that she did work on that ward, there were six deaths. Goldacre points out, "it seems odd that the death rate should go down on a ward at the precise moment that a serial killer – on a killing spree – arrives. If Lucia killed them all, then there must have been no natural deaths on that ward at all in the whole of the three years that she worked there."

Goldacre concludes, "the **prosecutors found seven deaths on one nurse's shifts**, in one hospital, in one city, in one country, in the world and **then drew a target around them**. This breaks a cardinal rule of any research involving statistics: you cannot find your hypothesis in your results" (Goldacre 2011).

Conclusion

The conclusion is that randomness does not mean uniformity. There are irregularities in randomness. One cannot survey randomness until finding an irregularity, find an improbable hypothesis that would explain the irregularity, and claim evidence for the hypothesis, when, in fact, randomness itself may adequately explain the irregularity.

References

Bender, A. P., Williams, A. N., Johnson, R. A., & Jagger, H. G. (1990). Appropriate Public Health Responses To Clusters: The Art Of Being Responsibly Responsive. American Journal of Epidemiology,132(Supp1), 48-52. doi:10.1093/oxfordjournals.aje.a115788

Bhatia, A., & Munroe, R. (2012, December 21). What does randomness look like? Retrieved July 07, 2017, from https://www.wired.com/2012/12/what-does-randomness-look-like/

Boland, P. J., & Hutchinson, K. (2000). Student Selection of Random Digits. Journal of the Royal Statistical Society: Series D (The Statistician),49(4), 519-529. doi:10.1111/1467-9884.00250

Caldwell, G. G. (1990). Twenty-Two Years Of Cancer Cluster Investigations At The Centers For Disease Control. American Journal of Epidemiology,132(Supp1), 43-47. doi:10.1093/oxfordjournals.aje.a115787

Cancer Clusters. (n.d.). Retrieved July 09, 2017, from https://www.cancer.org/cancer/cancer-causes/general-info/cancer-clusters.html

Datskovskiy, S. (n.d.). Man vs. Machine. Retrieved July 06, 2017, from http://www.loper-os.org/bad-at-entropy/manmach.html
Man vs. Machine Or, why Man is not a Particularly Good Source of Entropy

Feller, W. (1968). An introduction to probability theory and its applications. New York: John Wiley & Sons.

Figurska, M., Stańczyk, M., & Kulesza, K. (2008). Humans cannot consciously generate random numbers sequences: Polemic study. Medical Hypotheses,70(1), 182-185. doi:10.1016/j.mehy.2007.06.038

Gilovich, T. (2013). Heuristics and biases: the psychology of intuitive judgment. Cambridge: Cambridge University Press.

Gilovich, T., Vallone, R., & Tversky, A. (1985). The Hot Hand in Basketball: On the Misperception of Random Sequences. Cognitive Psychology,17, 295-314. doi:10.1017/cbo9780511808098.035

Goldacre, B. (2011). Bad science: quacks, hacks, and big pharma flacks. Toronto: Emblem Editions.

Gould, S. J. (2001). Bully for brontosaurus. London: Vintage.

Kahneman, D. (2015). *Thinking, fast and slow*. New York: Farrar, Straus and Giroux.

Orlin, B. (2013, November 11). The Patterns in the Stonework. Retrieved July 06, 2017, from https://mathwithbaddrawings.com/2013/11/11/the-patterns-in-the-stonework/

Pinker, S. (2012). The better angels of our nature: why violence has declined. NY, NY: Penguin Books.

Trumbo, C. (august 2000). Public Requests for Cancer Cluster Investigations: A Survey of State Health Departments. American Journal of Public Health,90(8), 1300-1302. Retrieved July 9, 2017.

Wagenaar, W. (1970). Subjective randomness and the capacity to generate information. Acta Psychologica,33, 233-242. doi:10.1016/0001-6918(70)90135-6

Further Reading

Gilovich, T. (2013). Heuristics and biases: the psychology of intuitive judgment. Cambridge: Cambridge University Press.

Goldacre, B. (2011). Bad science: quacks, hacks, and big pharma flacks. Toronto: Emblem Editions.

Kahneman, D. (2015). *Thinking, fast and slow*. New York: Farrar, Straus and Giroux.

Chapter 19: Normal Curve and Its Implications

Normal Curve and Its Implications

Normal Curve

The normal curve, also known as the bell curve and the Gaussian curve, models the distribution of many parameters including people's heights, IQ scores, blood pressures, body temperatures, and even the dates on which the swallows return to Capistrano! The normal curve plots the values of a parameter along the x-axis and the frequency of that parameter along the y-axis (Centers for Disease Control US Government 2012, see Fig. 19.1 below).

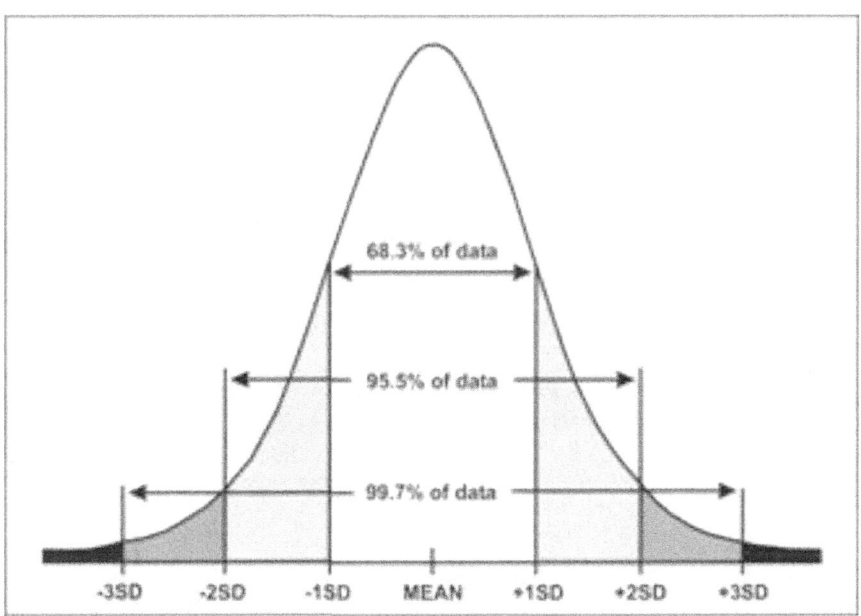

Fig. 19.1. Gaussian curve with standard deviations.

The configuration of the **normal curve is described by its mean and standard deviation**. The **mean** indicates where along the x-axis the center of the normal curve rests. The **standard deviation** indicates how closely around the mean the values cluster.

The area within one standard deviation on either side of the mean contains 68.3 percent of the values, within two standard deviations contains 95.5 percent of the values, and within three standard deviations contains 99.7 percent of the values.

The normal curve helps define **reference ranges**. The definition process consists in taking a large random sample from a population of healthy individuals, letting the values fall into their places in the normal distribution, and ***defining* the reference range as two standard deviations on either side of the mean** i.e., including 95.5 per cent of the population (UCSD Lab Medicine 2010, see below. Fig. 19.2)

For example, a lab report states that a patient's serum potassium is 4.1 with a reference range for this lab of 3.5-5.1. This report is indicating that the patient's serum potassium is 4.1 and that 95.5 percent of the healthy population has a serum potassium in the range 3.5-5.1.

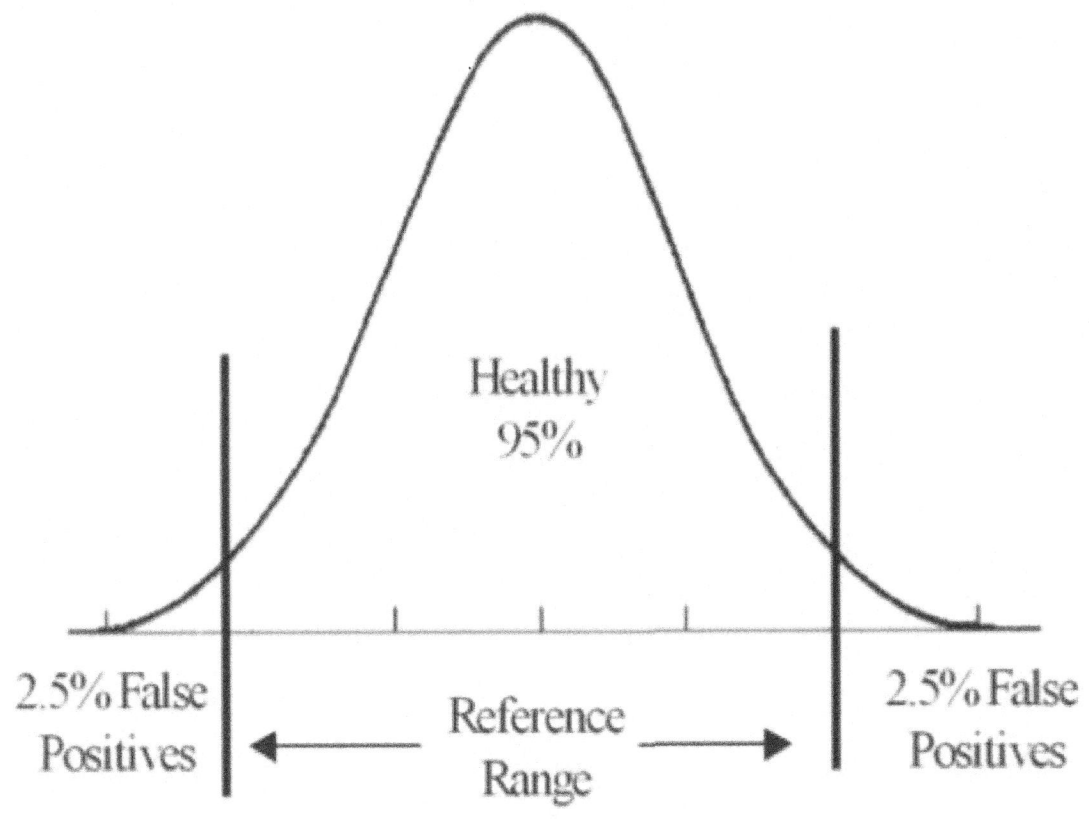

Fig. 19.2 Gaussian curve with reference range.

Null Hypothesis

So far, we know that our patient's serum potassium is 4.1 and that 95.5% of the healthy population falls within the range 3.5-5.1. The ready **inference** is **that** our patient is "normal" or "healthy" since he fell within the reference range. However, this inference is invalid. It **is flawed by** the previously described fallacy of **affirming the consequent** (see Chapter 14) and it is just as illogical as asserting that because streptococcal pharyngitis manifests as a sore throat, then a sore throat must mean streptococcal pharyngitis.

Nevertheless, the **inference that is justified is that we *cannot* say with a 95.5% level of confidence** that there is *no* difference between our patient and healthy people, **that our patient is *not* healthy**. Our patient may be healthy, or he may be unhealthy with offsetting conditions, for example, concomitant treatment with thiazide diuretics and potassium sparing diuretics, or diabetic acidosis and vomiting. In other words, we cannot reject the null hypothesis.

So, why this talk of the null hypothesis? The story begins in 1935 when the Austrian-English philosopher of science Karl Popper, authored the book *Logik der Forschung*. Hutchinson and Company first published Popper's book in English in 1959 as *The Logic of Scientific Discovery*.

In the book, Popper concerned himself with the problems of induction, or reasoning from the particular to the general. David Hume (1711-1776) first raised these problems when he questioned the validity of drawing conclusions inductively. He reasoned that induction was intrinsically different from deduction and so could not be justified by deduction. He also argued that induction could not be justified by experience, since experience itself was induction and, hence, begged the question (see Chapter 15).

Popper developed the idea that induction could not be justified by experience and argued that the observation of no number of white swans, however large, justifies the conclusion that all swans are white (Popper 2002, p 4).

Popper argued very influentially that science cannot seek to "prove" hypotheses by induction, but, rather, could only attempt to find evidence against them (Popper 2002, p 18). This concept gave birth to the notion of *attempting to reject the null hypothesis*. Finally, this concept explains why the range of **two standard deviations on either side of the mean is more accurately called the "reference range" than the "normal range."** Falling within this range is no proof of normalcy!

Problem of False Positives

By definition, **the 2.5 percent of the healthy population at each "tail" of the normal curve are** *defined* as abnormal or out of the reference range, even though they are healthy. They are, therefore, **false positives**.

These false positives are a reasonable price accepted for being able to identify a vast number of cases that lie outside the reference range *because they are* pathological and are true positives. This is especially true when

- The false positives do not receive potentially harmful treatment since they have no other corroborating studies and are asymptomatic. In other words, we have determined to "treat the patient not the test."
- The number of true positives actually is large compared to the number of false positives. If the number of false positives starts approaching the number of true positives, the utility of the test declines.

Thus far, we have discussed false positives in a single test. The next problem is the possibility of a false positive in a multi-test panel.

In a panel consisting of 20 independent tests, the chance of a healthy person testing within the reference range on all twenty tests is $0.95^{20} = 0.36$. Of course, the chance of one false positive is really not so high as $1.00 - 0.36 = 0.64$, since in a typical panel the individual parameters tested are not completely independent. However, it is evident that **a multi-test panel demonstrates a significant probability of reporting at least one false positive**.

The approach to a positive result on a multi-test panel is similar to that of a positive result on a single test, namely, investigation for symptomatology and corroboration with independent studies before institution of any potentially harmful treatment.

Physical vs. Statistical False Positives

The physical vs. statistical interplay in false positives is interesting. The temptation is to think that false positives must be due to equipment error or operator error, and, surely, sometimes this is the case. However, expensive equipment and decently paid technicians would not last long with a 4.5% error rate. The fact remains that **even with perfect equipment and operators, false positives occur as a statistical consequence of the test**. Further, statistically, more false positives will occur just outside the reference range than farther outside the reference range.

In accordance with the tendency to blame false positives on equipment or operator error, is the tendency to repeat the test, often in the expectation that the result will be vastly different. This is usually not the case. Certainly, repeated measurements of the same sample with the same equipment and same technician will produce another normal curve, but the standard deviation of this curve will be small and the repeated test will not likely differ markedly from the original.

Therapeutic or Replacement Levels

The normal curve finds another application in the area of therapeutic levels of drugs and replacement levels of deficient endogenous substances.

It may seem reasonable to increase the dosage of a drug or replacement until the patient reaches the therapeutic or reference range, or even the midpoint of the therapeutic or reference range. However, *if the patient is not responding to treatment and not experiencing side effects of therapy*, understanding of the normal curve indicates that treatment or replacement should increase to the upper limit of the reference range to be sure that it is adequate for 97.5% of patients. **Treatment or replacement to the midpoint of the range will only be sufficient for 50% of patients**.

Regression to the Mean

Another consequence of the normal curve is regression to the mean.

Inspection of the normal curve reveals that there are few cases under the curve laterally toward the tails with progressively more cases when moving centrally and maximizing dead center at the mean. In other words, in any normally distributed population **there are many more cases near the mean than far from it**.

This seemingly innocent fact explains both the Sports Illustrated jinx and the tendency of people to believe in the effectiveness of inert or incorrect medical treatments.

The **Sports Illustrated jinx** consists in the observation that athletes or teams appearing on the magazine's cover frequently experience a disappointing subsequent season. Nevertheless, this is a statistical rather than a voodoo effect. The cover featured the athlete or team because their performance was exceptional, i.e., far from their mean. However, there are far more performances closer to the mean than remote from it. Consequently, it is **probable that their next performance or season will regress toward the mean**.

In the case of **inert or incorrect medical treatments, people frequently adopt them when their symptoms are exceptionally severe**. The patients use magnets for their psoriasis or antibiotics for their viral upper respiratory infection and **a few days later, their symptoms have regressed toward the mean**. Consequently, the patients are convinced that they saw with their own eyes how well the useless therapy worked!

Conclusion

Examination of the normal curve throws light on the fact that "normal" and "abnormal" are defined statistically based on utility but that this utility has limitations and must be considered in decision-making in concert with attention to presence of symptoms, corroborating studies, and frequency of pathology in the general population. Further, understanding of the normal curve provides guidance in effective treatment or replacement and gives insight into why inert or incorrect treatments seem to work.

References

Centers for Disease Control US Government. (2012, May 18). Section 7: Measures of Spread. Retrieved July 04, 2017, from https://www.cdc.gov/ophss/csels/dsepd/ss1978/lesson2/section7.html Figure 2

Popper, K. (2002). Popper: the logic of scientific discovery. London: Routledge Classics.

UCSD Lab Medicine. (2010, March). Retrieved July 04, 2017, from http://ucsdlabmed.wikidot.com/chapter-1

Chapter 20: Innumeracy and Frequency Format Bias

Innumeracy

"Innumeracy" is a word popularized by mathematician John Allen Paulos some years ago in his book by the same name (Paulos 1990). He describes this **mathematical illiteracy** in its various forms and illustrates its broad distribution. Mathematical illiteracy is, unfortunately, more respectable than verbal illiteracy and more widespread, even among educated people.

Here are some studies exemplifying innumeracy among otherwise well educated patients.

Bramwell Investigation

Ros Bramwell studied a group of 43 pregnant women, 40 companions who accompanied the pregnant women to the clinic, 42 midwives, and 41 obstetricians. The **investigators gave all subjects information about a population and a Down syndrome screening test and asked them to estimate the probability that a positive test meant that a baby from that population had Down syndrome**.

The information consisted in the suppositions that 1% of the babies in the population had Down syndrome, that the test is positive in 90% of babies with Down Syndrome and in 1% of healthy babies. The probability of a baby testing positive actually having Down syndrome was 47.6%.

The reasoning was as follows: Among 10,000 babies, 100 would have Down syndrome according to the baseline frequency in the population. Of these 100, 90% or 90 babies would test positive. Of the remaining 9,900 babies, 1% or 99 would test positive. Therefore, a total of 90 + 99 = 189 would test positive. Of these, 90 would actually be positive. Therefore, 90 of the 189 or 47.6% of the positive testers would have Down syndrome.

Nevertheless, 86% of the responses were wrong. Only 43% of the obstetricians got the right answer, 0% of the midwives, 9% of the pregnant women, and 15% of the patients' companions.

Worse yet, reminiscent of the previously cited (Chapter 4) Dunning-Kruger investigations (Kruger and Dunning 1999), Bramwell asked the subjects who gave incorrect answers to rate confidence in their answers on a scale of 1 (not at all confident) to 6 (very confident). Disturbingly, the number of subjects who gave incorrect answers but rated their confidence in that answer as above 4 was 30% for patients, 56% for companions, 41% for midwives, and 73% for obstetricians.

Sox Investigation

Colin Sox (Sox 2006) studied 1502 US pediatricians. He sent them a scenario of a five-month-old girl admitted to hospital with hacking cough and perioral cyanosis. He indicated to them that the girl was started on erythromycin and given a direct fluorescent antibody test of her sputum for pertussis. He further informed them that the **pre-test likelihood that she had pertussis was 30%, and that the test had a sensitivity of 50% and a specificity of 95%. He informed them that the test proved negative and asked them to estimate the probability that the patient had pertussis**.

Sox reported that the correct answer was 0.18 and the reasoning is as follows: The test sensitivity is 0.5, meaning that of the 0.30 probability of true positive, it will detect 0.15 and miss 0.15. However, the test was negative. Therefore, it sampled either the 0.15 probability of true positives missed by the test, or the 0.70 probability of true negatives. Therefore, the probability of a true positive is 0.15 / (0.70 + 0.15) = 0.18.

Nevertheless, of the 1502 pediatricians, only 80 gave the correct answer. More importantly, over 200 responded with a probability of 0.5, and about three quarters responded with a probability of 0.3 or greater. These probabilities were clearly impossible given that the pre-test probability was 0.3 and the subsequent test was negative.

Gigerenzer Investigation

Gerd Gigerenzer (Gigerenzer 2008) and colleagues at the Max Planck Institute in Berlin and the Dartmouth Medical School in Hanover, New Hampshire, **assembled as subjects 160 gynecologists and asked them the probability of a woman having breast cancer given this information:**

Assume that you conduct breast cancer screening using mammography. You know the following information about the women in this region:
  • The probability that a woman has breast cancer is 1% (prevalence).
  • If a woman has breast cancer, the probability that she tests positive is 90% (sensitivity).
  • If a woman does not have breast cancer, the probability that she nevertheless tests positive is 9% (false positive rate).

A woman tests positive. She wants to know from you whether this means that she has breast cancer for sure, or what the chances are.

The best answer is
     (A) The probability that she has breast cancer is about 81%.
     (B) Out of 10 women with a positive mammogram, about 9 have breast cancer.
     (C) Out of 10 women with a positive mammogram, about 1 has breast cancer.
     (D) The probability that she has breast cancer is about 1%.

The best answer is (C) about one in 10. Again, the reasoning is that the probability of a woman in the population having breast cancer is 0.01. Since the sensitivity of the test is 0.90, then the probability of a woman in the population testing truly positive is 0.01 x 0.90 = 0.009. However, the probability of a woman in the population *not* having breast cancer is 0.99. Since the false positive probability of the test is 0.09, then the probability of a woman in the population testing falsely positive is 0.99 x 0.09 = 0.089. Consequently, the probability of a woman in the population who tests positive truly having breast cancer is 0.009 / (0.009 + 0.089) = 0.009 / 0.098 = 0.092, i.e., a probability of slightly more than 9%, about 1 in 10.

Unfortunately, only 21% of the gynecologists gave the best answer. In fact, 60% chose (B) 9 out of 10. The chief concern is that, even skipping the calculations, the gynecologists were not alerted by the low prevalence and relatively high false positive rate. The prevalence of 0.01 and false positive rate of 0.09 should have raised a flag that the probability would be more like 1 out of 9 or 10.

Frequency Format Bias

Frequency Format Bias is a term used by Gerd Gigerenzer (Gigerenzer 1996) to describe the phenomenon whereby **information presented as natural frequencies is perceived as being of larger magnitude than the same information presented as probabilities and is also understood more clearly**.

The natural frequency format expresses rates as xxxx/10,000. The probability format expresses rates as xx.xx% or 0.xxxx/1. While there is no difference mathematically, there is a big difference psychologically.

Yamagishi Study and Greater Magnitude

Yamagishi's 1997 study used as subjects 52 University of Washington undergraduates. He presented them with hypothetical cancer death rates of "2,414 out of 10,000," "1,286 out of 10,000," "24.14 out of 100," and "12.86 out of 100." After the presentation of each statistic, he asked them to evaluate cancer death risk on a scale of 0 (no risk) to 25 (maximum possible risk). He found that participants rated cancer as riskier when it was described as `kills 1,286 out of 10,000 people' than as `kills 24.14 out of 100 people' (Yamagishi 1997).

Yamagishi hypothesized that the effect could be explained by the anchoring bias combined with base-rate neglect, both of which we discussed previously.

Slovic Study and Greater Magnitude

Paul Slovic and colleagues published a study evidencing how communication of information as natural frequencies promotes perception of greater magnitude than the same information communicated as probability.

The Slovic group, in 2000, investigated whether mental health experts were as susceptible as the University of Washington undergraduates to the effects of Frequency Format Bias.

Slovic showed forensic psychologists and psychiatrists case summaries of patients hospitalized with mental disorder and asked them to judge the likelihood that the patient would harm someone within six months after discharge from the hospital. He found that at any given level of likelihood, the **psychiatrists and psychologists judged a patient as posing higher risk if that likelihood was derived from a frequency scale (e.g., 10 out of 100) than if it was derived from a probability scale (e.g., 10%).**

Monty Hall Problem and Clarity of Understanding

The natural frequency format of information communication introduces greater clarity into a conundrum known as "The Monty Hall Problem."

The Monty Hall Problem

The Monty Hall problem appeared in a game show called "Let's Make a Deal" that debuted on American television in 1963 and ran for decades thereafter. The game show host and executive producer was Monty Hall.

The famous problem involved, in addition to Monty Hall, a contestant chosen from the audience, and three doors. Behind one of the doors was a brand new, glitzy automobile. Behind each of the other two doors was a gag prize of little value, e.g., a goat.

Monty Hall invited the contestant to choose one of the three doors and promised the contestant the yet unknown prize behind that door. Monty Hall, of course, knew, in advance, what was behind each of the three doors.

The interesting feature of the program was that once the contestant had chosen a door, Monty Hall did not open that door. Instead, Monty opened one of the doors hiding a gag prize. Monty then offered the contestant the choice of keeping the selected door or switching to the other still-closed door. The contestant then made the decision to keep or switch, all accompanied by wild screams of advice from the audience.

The problem was whether winning the car was made any more probable by the decision to keep or the decision to switch. The problem was hotly debated, with the most widely held opinion being that no difference existed between keeping or switching. The thinking behind the "no difference" opinion was that once Monty Hall opened one of the gag prize doors, the probability of winning switched from 0.33 for each of the three doors to 0.50 for each of the two remaining doors.

However, it is *always* better to switch. The reason is that when the contestant takes the stage, the probability of the car being behind each door is 0.33. Therefore, the probability of the car being behind any door he or she chooses is 0.33, while the probability of the car being behind one of the other two doors is 0.67. Those probabilities do not change. The 0.67 probability is shared between the two not-chosen doors. When Monty Hall opens one of them to reveal a gag-prize, the 0.67 probability remains with the other door. **By switching, the contestant doubles the probability of winning the car.**

Jeremy Jones wrote an online computer simulation of the problem. More than 800,000 plays of the simulation by online visitors at http://www.stayorswitch.com confirmed the above findings (Jones 2014).

The Problem Clarification

The solution to the Monty Hall Problem becomes more clear when the situation is cast in terms of natural frequencies rather than in terms of probabilities.

Gerd Gigerenzer describes the situation thusly, "The crucial step is to think of a number of contestants, not just one. Let us take three, who each pick a different door. Assume the car is behind door 2. The first contestant picks door 1. Monty's only option is to open door 3, and he offers the contestant the opportunity to switch. Switching to door 2 wins. The second contestant picks door 3. This time, Monty has to open door 1, and switching to door 2 again wins. Only the third contestant who picks door 2 will lose when switching" (Gigerenzer 2015, p 126).

HIV Problem and Clarity of Understanding

Now let us see how communication of information as natural frequencies introduces greater clarity into a problem concerning HIV.

The HIV Problem

The HIV problem is that of healthy male who tests positive for HIV. He is in no particular high-risk group and the probability of HIV in this population is only 0.01%. The test is 99.9% sensitive and 99.99% specific. What is the probability that this patient has HIV?

The first glance estimate is that this man most certainly has HIV.

The Problem Clarification

Gerd Gigerenzer then described the problem as a problem in Bayesian analysis and calculated that the probability of the man having HIV was 0.999/0.999 + 0.9999.

Gigerenzer then described the problem in natural frequencies. He said that of 10,000 such men, one would have HIV and would test positive for it. Of the other 9,999, none would have HIV but one would test positive for it. Therefore, the **probability of our patient having HIV would be 1/1+1 or 1 in 2** (Gigerenzer 2013).

The problem becomes much clearer when phrased in terms of natural frequencies.

Countermeasure to Innumeracy

Presentation of information in the **natural frequency format** facilitates understanding of potentially difficult numerical concepts. In this sense, it **can serve as a countermeasure to innumeracy**.

Countermeasure to Deceptive Comparisons

Presentation of information in the format of abstract probabilities seems to minimize the magnitude of that information.

Clearly, this presents the possibility of biased judgments when information in probability format is offered for comparison with information in natural frequency format. At least two lessons here present themselves.

First, if we wish our patients to be able to make decisions regarding medical or surgical interventions as clearly and unbiasedly as possible, we should **present** to them the **information on benefits and risks in the same terms, preferably as natural frequencies**.

Second, if, in examining the literature, we note that benefits are presented as natural frequencies while risks or harms are presented as probabilities, or vice versa, we should attempt to recast all parameters in terms of natural frequencies. Otherwise, **heterogeneous presentations can bias the appreciation of benefits vs. risks**.

Unfortunately, such heterogeneous presentation of benefits vs. risks or harms is not unusual in the literature. Sedrakyan and Shih studied articles published in the *British Medical Journal*, the *Journal of the American Medical Association*, and *The Lancet* from 2004 to 2006 and found this heterogeneous presentation in one of every three articles (Sedrakyan 2007).

Conclusion

Innumeracy, or mathematical illiteracy, is widespread, even among educated people. So too is frequency format bias whereby information presented as probabilities is perceived as being of smaller magnitude than the same information presented as probabilities. Finally, information presented as natural frequencies is understood more clearly than information presented as probabilities.

The two lessons here are: First, for optimum understanding, endeavor to present information in a natural frequency format. Second, in presenting comparisons, especially between risks and benefits, present all information in the same format, preferably natural frequencies.

References

Bramwell, West, & Salmon. (2006). Health professionals' and service users' interpretation of screening test results: Experimental study. *Brtitish Medical Journal,*284-286.

Gigerenzer, G. (1996). The Psychology of Good Judgment. *Medical Decision Making,16*(3), 273-280. doi:10.1177/0272989x9601600312

Gigerenzer, G. (2013). Better doctors, better patients, better decisions: envisioning health care 2020;. Cambridge, Mass.: MIT Press.

Gigerenzer, G. (2015). *Risk savvy: how to make good decisions.* London: Penguin Books.

Gigerenzer, G., Gaissmaier, W., Kurz-Milcke, E., Schwartz, L., & Woloshin, S. (2008). Helping Doctors and Patients Make Sense of Health Statistics. Psychological Science in the Public Interest,8(2), 53-96.

Jones, J. (2014). The Monty Hall Problem. Retrieved October 30, 2017, from http://www.stayorswitch.com/

Kruger, J., & Dunning, D. (1999). Unskilled and unaware of it: How difficulties in recognizing one's own incompetence lead to inflated self-assessments. *Journal of Personality and Social Psychology, 77*(6), 1121-1134. doi:10.1037//0022-3514.77.6.1121

Paulos, J. A. (1990). Innumeracy: Mathematical illiteracy and its consequences. New York: Vintage Books.

Sedrakyan, A., & Shih, C. (2007). Improving Depiction of Benefits and Harms. *Medical Care,45*(Suppl 2). doi:10.1097/mlr.0b013e3180642f69

Sox, C. M., Koepsell, T. D., Doctor, J. N., & Christakis, D. A. (2006). Pediatricians Clinical Decision Making. Archives of Pediatrics & Adolescent Medicine,160(5), 487. doi:10.1001/archpedi.160.5.487

Yamagishi, K. (1997). When a 12.86% mortality is more dangerous than 24.14%: implications for risk communication. Applied Cognitive Psychology,11(6), 495-506. doi:10.1002/(sici)1099-0720(199712)11:6<495::aid-acp481>3.0.co;2-j

Further Reading

Gigerenzer, G. (2013). Better doctors, better patients, better decisions: envisioning health care 2020;. Cambridge, Mass.: MIT Press.

Gigerenzer, G. (1996). The Psychology of Good Judgment. *Medical Decision Making,16*(3), 273-280. doi:10.1177/0272989x9601600312

Gigerenzer, G. (2015). *Risk savvy: how to make good decisions.* London: Penguin Books.

Gigerenzer, G., Gaissmaier, W., Kurz-Milcke, E., Schwartz, L., & Woloshin, S. (2008). Helping Doctors and Patients Make Sense of Health Statistics. Psychological Science in the Public Interest,8(2), 53-96.

Kruger, J., & Dunning, D. (1999). Unskilled and unaware of it: How difficulties in recognizing one's own incompetence lead to inflated self-assessments. *Journal of Personality and Social Psychology, 77*(6), 1121-1134. doi:10.1037//0022-3514.77.6.1121

Using Medical Tests

Chapter 21: Sensitivity, Specificity, and Likelihood Ratio

A CNN news release dated June 2, 2015 reported, "Airport screeners failed to detect explosives and weapons in nearly every test that an undercover team conducted at dozens of airports ... "red teams" with the Department of Homeland Security's Office of the Inspector General were able to get banned items through the screening process in 67 out of 70 tests it conducted across the nation" (Bradner 2015).

On the other hand, a 2003 CBS *60 Minutes* broadcast by Leslie Stahl reported, "The FBI has long maintained that fingerprint identification is an exact science that can be used to match prints with 100 percent certainty. But recently, the bureau was forced to admit that three top analysts all made the same mistake when they swore that fingerprint evidence linked Oregon lawyer Brandon Mayfield to the terrorist bombings in Madrid. Mayfield spent two weeks in jail before the FBI admitted its error and offered an apology" (Stahl 2003).

These two examples respectively describe failures to meet two of the most important criteria of tests, namely, sensitivity and specificity.

Sensitivity

Sensitivity is the proportion of true positives that are identified as positive by the test. It is the **true positive rate** of the test. Sensitivity is given by the formula

> Sensitivity = Test Positives / Real Positives
> = Test Positives / (Test Positives + Test False Negatives)
> = Probability of Positive Test in Person that Actually Has the Disease in the Population

Thus, the airport screeners mentioned above exhibited a sensitivity of only 3/70 or 4.3%. The time-honored fecal occult blood test (FOBT), when tested against colonoscopy, yielded a disappointing sensitivity of 76.5% for colorectal neoplasia and 69.2% for colorectal cancer (Niv 1995).

In terms of Venn diagrams, **99% sensitivity of a test can be visualized as follows:**

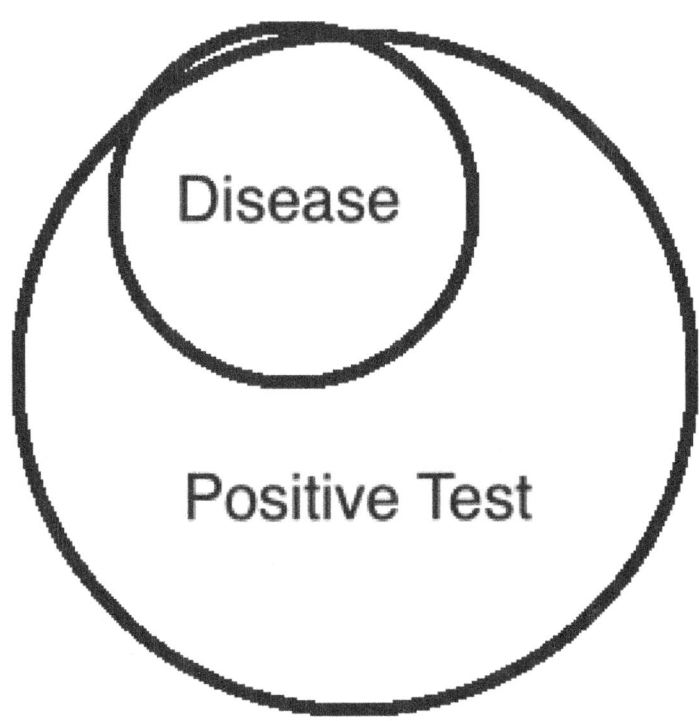

Fig. 21.1 Venn diagram of a highly sensitive test.

Here the outer circle represents the positive test and the inner circle represents presence of the disease. The test is 99% sensitive because very little of the disease escapes detection by the test. Notably, **however, this highly sensitive test may register a number of false positives**.

In the terms of symbolic logic, a 100% sensitive test is "implied" or "entailed" by the disease targeted by the test. Phrased another way, **a positive 100% sensitive test is a necessary condition for the presence of the disease tested for**. Phrased yet another way, in a 100% sensitive test, the presence of the disease is the *antecedent* and the positive test result is the *consequent,* so a negative test result proves the *absence* of the disease tested for by the method of *negating the consequent.*

Previously, Chapter 14 discussed how ***negating the consequent* is a valid inference**. The example cited was that since all cities in Illinois are cities in the US, and since Mumbai is not a city in the US, then Mumbai is not a city in Illinois.

Similarly, if all patients having a disease are positive on a given test and a specific patient tests negative, then that specific patient does not have the disease.

In the well-publicized O.J. Simpson trial of 1995, the prosecution offered the premise that the killer of Ronald Goldman and Nicole Brown Simpson wore a pair of bloody gloves found near the scene. Defense attorney Johnnie Cochran invoked the principle of negating the consequent with his famous dictum "If the gloves don't fit, you must acquit." Sure enough, the gloves did not fit O.J. Simpson and the jury acquitted Simpson of the murders.

This mode of reasoning from a 100% sensitive, or almost 100% sensitive, test by negating the consequent embodies itself in the **mnemonic "SNOUT" meaning "sensitivity negative rules out."**

Thus, when Chan studied 149 consecutive pregnant women with suspected deep vein thrombosis (DVT) and found that the SimpliRED D-dimer assay was 100% sensitive, he concluded, "The assay may be useful in pregnancy because a normal result excluded DVT" (Chan 2007).

Similarly, in Eisenhofer's study of the use of plasma free metanephrines in the diagnosis of pheochromocytoma, he concluded, "The high sensitivity of plasma free metanephrines means that a normal test result reliably excludes all but the smallest of pheochromocytomas so that no other tests are necessary" (Eisenhofer 2000).

Specificity

Specificity is the proportion of true negatives that are identified as negative by the test. It is the **true negative rate**. Specificity is given by the formula

Specificity = Test Negatives / Real Negatives
= Test Negatives / (Test Negatives + Test False Positives)
= Probability of Negative Test in Person without the Disease in the Population

Thus, the FBI fingerprint lab mentioned above "maintained that fingerprint identification is an exact science that can be used to match prints with 100 percent certainty," consequently, it claimed a specificity of 100%. Less spectacularly, the fecal occult blood test (FOBT), when tested against colonoscopy, yielded a disappointing specificity of 56.7% for colorectal neoplasia and 73.2% for colorectal cancer (Niv 1995).

In terms of Venn diagrams, 99% specificity of a test can be visualized as follows:

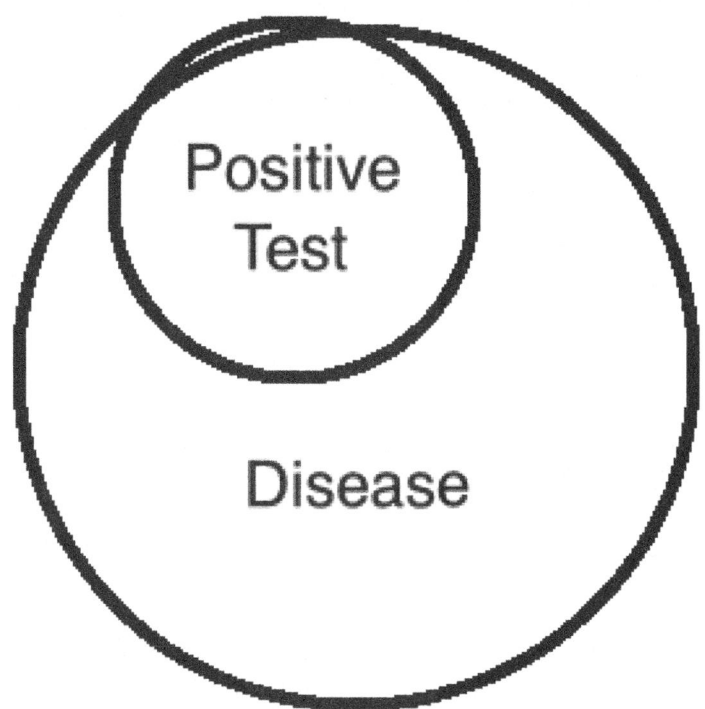

Fig. 21.2 Venn diagram of a highly specific test.

Here the inner circle represents the positive test and the outer circle represents presence of the disease. The test is 99% specific because almost every positive test identifies a presence of the disease. Notably, however, this **highly specific test may register a number of false negatives.**

Previously, Chapter 14 discussed how *affirming the antecedent* is a valid inference. The example cited was that since all cities in Illinois are cities in the US, and since Chicago is a city in Illinois, then, Chicago is a city in the US. Similarly, if all patients testing positive have the disease and this specific patient tests positive, then this specific patient has the disease.

This mode of reasoning from a 100% specific, or almost 100% specific, test by affirming the antecedent embodies itself in the **mnemonic "SPIN" meaning "specificity positive rules in."**

Thus, when Willmann's study compared 16-detector row CT angiography against digital subtraction angiography in the assessment of aortoiliac and lower extremity arteries in patients with peripheral arterial disease, and it found a 97% specificity (Willmann 2005), it lent very strong support to the inference that a stenosis discovered on 16-detector CT angiography, would also be evident on digital subtraction angiography.

Pathognomonic signs or symptoms are those with an extremely high specificity, whether their sensitivity is high or low. Their presence virtually assures the presence of a disease or condition. Textbooks of physical diagnosis are replete with **examples of such signs or symptoms**:

- Reed–Sternberg cells for Hodgkins lymphoma
- Trousseau sign and Chvostek sign for hypocalcemia
- Koplik spots for measles
- Kayser-Fleischer ring for Wilson's disease
- Pharyngeal pseudomembrane for diphtheria
- Grey-Turner sign for hemorrhagic pancreatitis
- Rice-water stool for cholera
- Kernig sign and Brudzinski sign for meningitis
- Machine-like murmur for patent ductus arteriosis
- Pill-rolling tremor for Parkinson disease
- Auer rods for acute myeloid leukemia
- Aschoff bodies for rheumatic fever
- Negri bodies for rabies
- Tophi for gout
- Yellow or green vision for digoxin toxicity

Likelihood Ratio

Positive Likelihood Ratio LR+

Another parameter useful in test applications is the **positive likelihood ratio (LR+)**. The LR+ describes for a given test result, how many times more or less likely are patients with a particular disease to have that test result than patients without the disease. It is the ratio of the probability of that test result in people who have the disease to the probability in people who do not have the disease (Deeks 2004). Put more simply, **the LR+ tells how the odds of the disease increase when the test is positive** (Simon n.d.).

.

The positive likelihood ratio is given by the formula

$$LR+ = sensitivity / (1 - specificity)$$

As an LR+ increases from 1.0 to infinity, it increasingly supports the diagnosis of interest. As an LR+ decreases from 1.0 to 0.0, it increasingly militates against the diagnosis of interest. An LR+ of 1.0 is neither confirmatory nor disconfirmatory (McGee 2002).

Importantly, a **positive likelihood ratio above 10 for a diagnostic test is considered to be strong evidence to "rule in" disease** (Jaeschke 2002).

Negative Likelihood Ratio LR-

On the other hand, the **negative likelihood ratio (LR-)** describes, for a given test result, how many times more or less likely persons without a particular disease are to have that test result than persons with the disease. It is the ratio of the probability of that test result in people without the disease to the probability in people who do have the disease. Put more simply, **the LR- tells how the odds of the disease decrease when the test is negative** (Simon n.d.).

The negative likelihood ratio is given by the formula

LR- = (1- sensitivity) / specificity

As an LR- increases from 1.0 to infinity, it increasingly supports absence of the diagnosis of interest. As an LR- decreases from 1.0 to 0.0, it increasingly militates against absence of the diagnosis of interest. An LR- of 1.0 is neither confirmatory nor disconfirmatory.

Finally, a **negative likelihood ratio below 0.1 is considered sufficient evidence to "rule out" disease** (Jaeschke 2002).

LR+/LR-

Jekel succinctly explains the relationship between LR+ and LR-. He cites the formulas

LR+ = sensitivity / (1 – specificity)
LR- = (1- sensitivity) / specificity

and indicates that since a useful test should have high sensitivity and high specificity, **the LR+ should be high and the LR- should be low**. Expressing this quantitatively, many consider an **LR+/LR- ratio < 50 to be indicative of a weak test** (Jekel 2007, p. 110).

Prostate Specific Antigen (PSA) Example

Holstrom's group studied the usefulness of prostate specific antigen (PSA) as a screening test in predicting subsequent diagnosis of prostate cancer in 540 prostate cancer cases and 1034 age and date-of-blood-draw matched controls.

The **group calculated the sensitivity, specificity, and likelihood ratios of PSA at several concentrations** (Holstrom 2009).
For various PSA levels, the likelihood ratios were as follows:

PSA Level (ng/ml)	LR+	LR-
0.5	1.15	0.04
1.0	1.73	0.08
2.0	3.15	0.30
5.0	6.35	0.70
10.0	12.34	0.88
20.0	28.11	0.95

Table 21.1 PSA concentrations vs. likelihood ratios. After Holstrom, "Prostate specific antigen for early detection of prostate cancer: longitudinal study" in the *British Medical Journal*, September 2009.

Using Jaeschke's criteria of LR+ > 10 to "rule in" and LR- < 0.1 to "rule out," it was evident that a **PSA level <1.0 virtually ruled out a diagnosis of prostate cancer** during the follow-up period (Holstrom 2009). This is certainly consistent with the current use of PSA to militate against recurrence of prostate cancer after treatment.

On the other hand, using Jaeschke's criteria, a **PSA level > 10.0 is highly suggestive of prostate cancer**. However, this level had sensitivity < 0.13, meaning that it would overlook too many prostate cancers to be useful in screening.

The LR+/LR- ratio for the 1.0 ng/ml PSA level is 21.9 and, for the 10.0 ng/ml level, it is 14.02. The LR+/LR- ratio for the 20.0 ng/ml level is 29.59. All are below the threshold of 50 used as a criterion for useful tests.

Calculating Post-Test Probability from LR and Pre-Test Odds

This method begins with sensitivity and specificity to determine likelihood ratio. It then applies likelihood ratio to pre-test odds to determine post-test odds. Finally, it converts post-test odds to post-test probability.

As stated above,

LR+ = sensitivity / (1 – specificity)
LR- = (1- sensitivity) / specificity

Pre-test odds are stated as a ratio. For example, if condition A affects 7% of a certain population, then the pre-test odds of A in that population are 7 / 93. If a given test has an LR+ of 15, then

Post-Test Odds = Pre-Test Odds x Likelihood Ratio (Simon)
$$= (7 / 93) \times 15$$
$$= 105 / 93$$
$$= 1.129$$

Then

Post-Test Probability = Post-Test Odds / Post-Test Odds + 1
$$= 1.129 / 2.129$$
$$= 0.530$$

Serum Ferritin Example

Consider this example from the Centre for Evidence-Based Medicine at Oxford University (Likelihood Ratios 2016). The example concerns **serum ferritin as a diagnostic test for iron deficiency anemia** carried out on 2579 patients (assume all are premenopausal females). Suppose that for a serum ferritin level within a certain range, the sensitivity for iron deficiency anemia is 90% and the specificity is 85%.

LR+ = sens / (1-spec) = 90/15 = **6**
LR- = (1-sens) / (spec) = 10/85 = **0.12**

Further, in the population of premenopausal females in North America, the **baseline probability of having iron deficiency anemia is about 5%** (Harper 2017); and, the pre-test odds are therefore 0.05 / 0.95 = 0.0526.

But,
Post-Test Odds = Pre-Test Odds x Likelihood Ratio

Consequently, the odds for a patient positive with this test result are approximately 6 x 0.0526 = 0.316.

However,
Post-Test Probability = Post-Test Odds / Post-Test Odds + 1

So,
Post-Test Probability = 0.316 / 1.316
$$= 0.24$$
$$= 24\%$$

On the other hand, the LR- of 0.12 indicates that the odds of a patient with this level of serum ferritin not having iron deficiency anemia are 0.12 times that of a person in the baseline population. Further, in the baseline population of premenopausal females in North America, the odds of not having iron deficiency anemia are 0.95 / 0.05 = 19. Consequently, the **odds for a patient negative with this test result not having iron deficiency anemia are approximately 0.12 x 19 = 2.28**.

But,

$$\text{Post-Test Probability} = \text{Post-Test Odds} / \text{Post-Test Odds} + 1$$

So,

Post-Test Probability = 2.28 / 3.28
= 0.695
= 70%

If these probabilities are not so convincing as one might have hoped, it should be borne in mind that the LR+/LR- ratio here (6.0 / 0.12) is only 50.

Fagan's Nomogram of Post-Test Probabilities from Likelihood Ratios and Pre-Test Probabilities

The serum ferritin example reveals a difficulty in using the "LR and Pre-Test Odds" method of computing post-test probabilities. This method uses sensitivity and specificity to determine likelihood ratio, applying likelihood ratio to pre-test odds to determine post-test odds, and then the conversion of post-test odds to post-test probability.

T.J. Fagan published in *New England Journal of Medicine* (Fagan 1975) a **nomogram (see below) that begins with pre-test probability, applies the likelihood ratio, and outputs post-test probability.** Fagan's nomogram is logarithmic and executes multiplication by transforming it into addition.

Using the nomogram consists simply in selecting the point on the vertical line labeled "pre-test probability" (prevalence), then selecting the point on the vertical line labeled "likelihood ratio," next connecting the points with a straight line, and, finally, extending that line until it crosses the vertical line labeled "post-test probability." The situation is similar for LR+ and LR-.

Fagan's nomogram is conveniently available as a smart phone app.

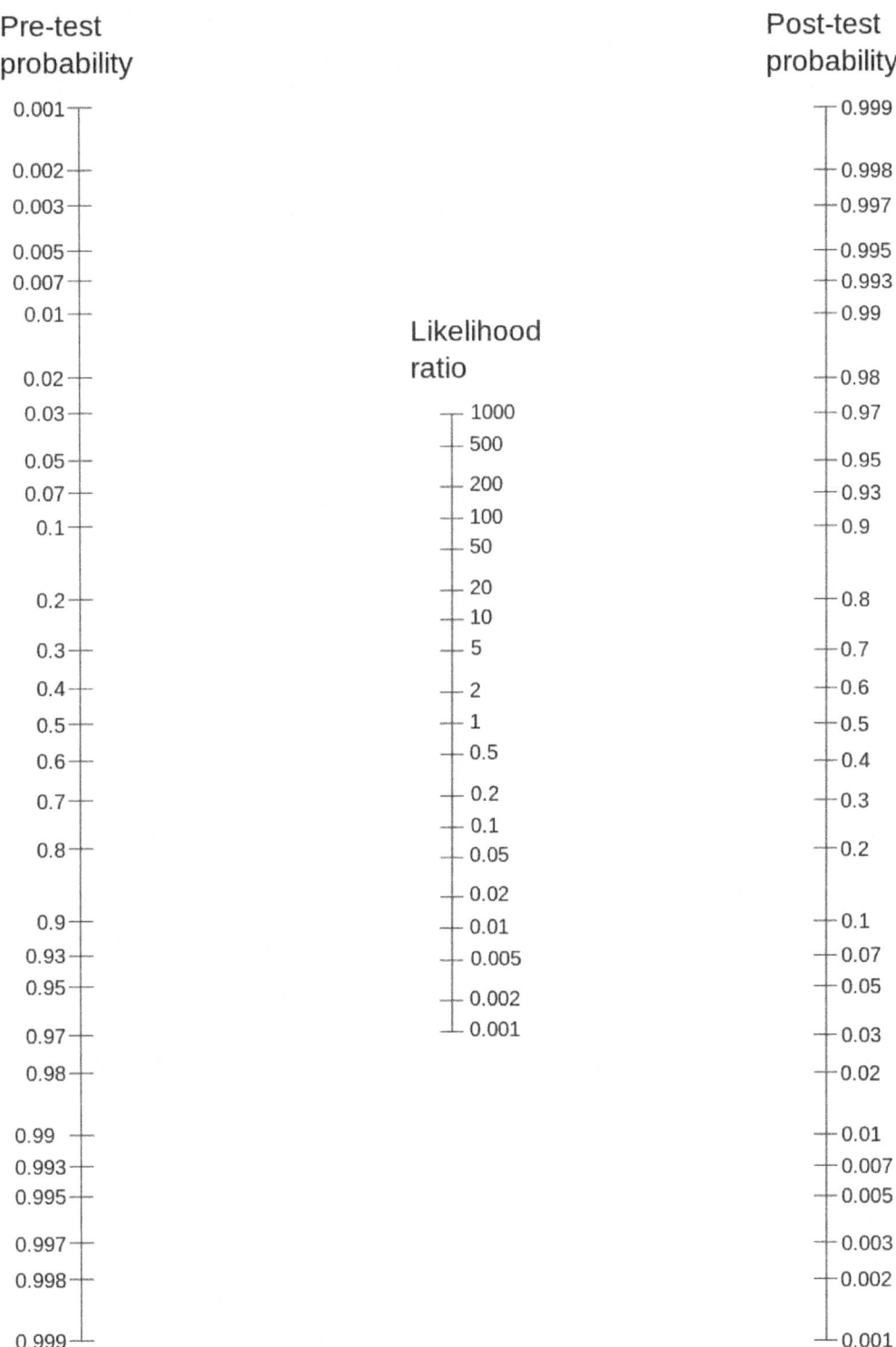

Fig. 21.3 Fagan's nomogram.

McGee's Estimates of Post-Test Probabilities from Likelihood Ratios and Pre-Test Probabilities

Like Fagan, McGee also **begins with pre-test probability, applies the likelihood ratio, and ends with post-test probability. However, McGee dispenses with the nomogram and produces an** *estimate* **of the post-test probability** *change*.

McGee provides a table of 13 estimates of post-test probability changes that are useful at the bedside. His estimates are accurate to within 10% of the calculated answer when pre-test probabilities are between 10% and 90% (McGee 2002). The easiest, LRs to remember are 2, 5, and 10 along with 0.1, 0.2, and 0.5.

Likelihood Ratio	Approximate Probability Change %
0.1	-45
0.2	-30
0.5	-15
2	15
5	30
10	45

Table 21.2 Likelihood ratios vs. approximate probability changes. After McGee, "Simplifying Likelihood Ratios," *Journal of General Internal Medicine,* August 2002.

The Relevance of Prevalence

The prevalence, pre-test probability, or base-rate, is of critical importance in deciding to apply the likelihood ratio. **With an extremely low or high pre-test probability, a likelihood ratio may not make substantial difference. With a mid-range pre-test probability, likelihood ratio may change a risk significantly.**

For example, let us take again a LR+ of 6. With an LR+ of 6 and a pre-test probability of 0.01 (1%), the post-test probability becomes 0.056 (5.6%). With an LR+ of 6 and a pre-test probability of 0.99 (99%), the post-test probability becomes 0.9983 (99.8%).

Nevertheless, with a pre-test probability of 20%, the post-test probability becomes 60%.
A difference in probability between 1% and 5.6% or between 99.0% and 99.8% may make no difference in clinical decision-making. However, a difference in probability between 20% and 60% might make a difference between accepting and rejecting a dangerous intervention.

Indefinite Prevalence

Nevertheless, **prevalence in a relevant population, unlike sensitivity and specificity of a test, may be difficult to obtain**. The reason is that developing prevalence information demands extensive human and monetary resources. Such resources are likely to be allotted only if the information applies to large populations, such as the residents of a country or a state or province. Consequently, the local prevalence information required to treat specific patients in a specific demographic may be sparse.

When local prevalence information is sparse, two options are possible.

First option is to limit decision-making to the information provided by the LR+ and LR- alone. In the context of the aforementioned iron deficiency example, this option consists of ending with the conclusion that the serum ferritin level suggests the probability of the patient's having iron deficiency anemia is six times that of the general population. Further inferences are not attempted.

Second option is to apply the LRs to an *estimate* of the prevalence of the condition locally. This estimate could be an adjustment from a baseline national prevalence. MedicalHomePortal.org publishes prevalence data on children in family practices in the US (Diagnosis Prevalence List 2017). Additionally, the Centers for Disease Control (CDC) publishes data on disease prevalence at www.cdc.gov/DataStatistics (Data & Statistics | CDC 2017). The presence of risk factors might further adjust a baseline estimate. Although such estimates and adjustments are imprecise, they may be the best practical option.

Finally, in the above examples for sensitivity and specificity, we have simplified the issue, using average values for these parameters. **Technically, however, sensitivity and specificity each has its own range with a 95% confidence interval**, sometimes indicated as such. In these cases, it is appropriate to calculate LRs for the high and low limits of the confidence interval to determine the confidence intervals of the LRs.

Conclusion

The common belief is that tests provide conclusions: "What did my test show, Doctor?" However, the fact is that **tests simply provide information**. The reliability and applicability of that information is always open to question. Selection of the right test, for the right patient, at the right time, in the right context, with the right analysis of results, determines the utility of the test.

References

Bradner, E., & Marsh, R. (2015, June 02). TSA screeners failed tests to detect explosives, weapons - CNNPolitics. Retrieved September 18, 2017, from http://www.cnn.com/2015/06/01/politics/tsa-failed-undercover-airport-screening-tests/index.html

Chan, W., Chunilal, S., Lee, A., Crowther, M., Rodger, M., & Ginsberg, J. S. (2007). A Red Blood Cell Agglutination d-Dimer Test to Exclude Deep Venous Thrombosis in Pregnancy. *Annals of Internal Medicine,147*(3), 165. doi:10.7326/0003-4819-147-3-200708070-00005

Data & Statistics | CDC. (2017, September 27). Retrieved October 01, 2017, from https://www.cdc.gov/DataStatistics/

Deeks, J. J. (2004). Diagnostic tests 4: likelihood ratios. Bmj,329(7458), 168-169. doi:10.1136/bmj.329.7458.168

Diagnosis Prevalence List. (n.d.). Retrieved October 01, 2017, from https://www.medicalhomeportal.org/diagnoses-and-conditions/diagnosis-prevalence-list

Eisenhofer, G., Walther, M., Keiser, H., Lenders, J., Friberg, P., & Pacak, K. (2000). Plasma metanephrines: a novel and cost-effective test for pheochromocytoma. *Brazilian Journal of Medical and Biological Research,33*(10), 1157-1169. doi:10.1590/s0100-879x2000001000005

Fagan, T. (1975). Nomogram for Bayess Theorem. *New England Journal of Medicine,293*(5), 257-257. doi:10.1056/nejm197507312930513

Harper, J. (2017, July 03). Iron Deficiency Anemia. Retrieved September 29, 2017, from http://emedicine.medscape.com/article/202333-overview

Holmstrom, B., Johansson, M., Bergh, A., Stenman, U., Hallmans, G., & Stattin, P. (2009). Prostate specific antigen for early detection of prostate cancer: longitudinal study. *Bmj,339*(Sep24 1). doi:10.1136/bmj.b3537

https://www.cdc.gov/datastatistics/index.html

Jaeschke, R., Guyatt, G., & Lijmer, J. (2002). Diagnostic Tests. In *Users' guides to the medical literature.*(pp. 121-140). Chicago, IL: AMA Press.

Jekel, J. (1996). *Epidemiology, biostatistics, and preventative medicine. WB Saunders, 1996*. WB Saunders.

Jekel, J. F. (2007). *Epidemiology, biostatistics, and preventive medicine.* Philadelphia: Saunders/Elsevier.

Likelihood Ratios. (2016, March 07). Retrieved September 29, 2017, from http://www.cebm.net/likelihood-ratios/

Lower Extremity Arteries Assessed with 16–Detector Row CT Angiography: Prospective Comparison with Digital Subtraction Angiography. *Radiology,236*(3), 1083-1093. doi:10.1148/radiol.2362040895

Mcgee, S. (2002). Simplifying likelihood ratios. *Journal of General Internal Medicine,17*(8), 647-650. doi:10.1046/j.1525-1497.2002.10750.x

Niv, Y., & Sperber, A. (1995). Sensitivity, specificity, and predictive value of fecal occult blood testing. Am J Gastroenterol,90(11), 1974-1977 . Retrieved September 18, 2017.

Stahl, Lesley . "Fingerprints: Infallible Evidence? ." 60 Minutes, CBS, 16 July 2003.

Simon, S. (n.d.). P.Mean: Main page for the P.Mean website (created 2008-06-21). Retrieved March 06, 2018, from http://www.pmean.com/

Willmann, J. K., Baumert, B., Schertler, T., Wildermuth, S., Pfammatter, T., Verdun, F. R., . . . Böhm, T. (2005). Aortoiliac and Lower Extremity Arteries Assessed with 16–Detector Row CT Angiography: Prospective Comparison with Digital Subtraction Angiography. *Radiology,236*(3), 1083-1093. doi:10.1148/radiol.2362040895

Further Reading

Holmstrom, B., Johansson, M., Bergh, A., Stenman, U., Hallmans, G., & Stattin, P. (2009). Prostate specific antigen for early detection of prostate cancer: longitudinal study. *Bmj,339*(Sep24 1). doi:10.1136/bmj.b3537

Mcgee, S. (2002). Simplifying likelihood ratios. *Journal of General Internal Medicine,17*(8), 647-650. doi:10.1046/j.1525-1497.2002.10750.x

Chapter 22: Diagnostic and Screening Tests

Diagnostic and Screening Tests

Medical tests fall into the two broad categories: **diagnostic** and **screening**.

A **diagnostic test is used when a patient is complaining of symptoms or exhibiting clinical signs**. Thus, consider a patient who presents to the dermatologist with a skin lesion that is asymmetric, has irregular borders, is multicolored, and is three-eighths inch in diameter. The dermatologist does a biopsy, perhaps excisional, to determine if the lesion is a malignant melanoma. The biopsy is a diagnostic test.

A **screening test is used when a member of the public is not complaining of symptoms or exhibiting clinical signs**. Consider a scene at the local mall where a shopper passes a local hospital's health fair that is offering free blood pressure measurements and the shopper has himself tested. The shopper is not complaining of symptoms or exhibiting clinical signs. Consequently, the blood pressure measurement is a screening test.

Some tests are *only diagnostic*. Such would be the case of the excisional biopsy above, since one would not do this procedure on normal appearing skin in a patient without signs or symptoms.

However, **some tests can be *diagnostic or screening*** depending upon the circumstances. The blood pressure measurement is a screening test when the shopper casually has his blood pressure measured at the mall health fair. Nevertheless, the blood pressure measurement is a diagnostic test when the patient experiences nosebleeds and headaches and his physician measures his blood pressure in consideration of the diagnosis of hypertension.

Screening

Again, excisional biopsies on the normal-appearing skin of persons without symptoms or clinical signs of disease are inappropriate. However, when tests are cheap, painless, and noninvasive, the temptation may arise to test everyone. Nevertheless, there is a **major error in assuming that any test that is cheap, painless, and noninvasive, especially if it is useful in diagnosis, would also be helpful in screening**.

The problem is that a real-world test, i.e., one with less than perfect specificity, identifies some false positives. When that test is applied to a population in which the number of true positives compares favorably with the number of false positives, the existence of false positives may be tolerable. A test is used in such a way when the test is used **diagnostically**, that is, when the patient exhibits symptoms, signs, or some evidence of having the disease.

On the other hand, when the same test is applied for **screening**, it is applied to a broad population, without symptoms or signs. This population has a much smaller percentage of true positives than a population of patients who are symptomatic. However, the specificity of the test is the same. It still identifies the same *percentage of tested persons* as false positives, but this time the number of tested persons is the much larger asymptomatic population rather than the much smaller number of symptomatic persons. This leads to a large number of false positive identifications.

Subsequently, **confirming or disconfirming these (mostly false) positives requires asymptomatic persons to have further testing or procedures, at additional expense and risk of injury**. This is superimposed upon the initial expense and risk of the original screening. Finally, false positives, especially when clumsily communicated to the patient, can be a source of considerable distress.

Prostate Specific Antigen (PSA) Example

An example of a test of doubtful use in screening is the prostate specific antigen (PSA) test. Until recently, this test was widely used in screening for prostate cancer. Lately, however, **the test has lost favor because of false positives, inability to identify the small number of prostate cancers that are aggressive, harms of overdiagnosis, and complications of overtreatment**.

According to the National Institute of Health, National Cancer Institute, Division of Cancer Prevention, for every 1000 men screened with a PSA test, 100-120 will get a false positive result that will lead to anxiety and, more importantly, to biopsy. One-third of the men biopsied would experience infection, pain, or bleeding. An additional 110 will have treatment, of whom at least 50 men will have complications: erectile dysfunction in 29 men, urinary incontinence in 18 men, serious cardiovascular events in 2 men, deep vein thrombosis or pulmonary embolism in 1 man, and death due to the treatment in less than 1 man (Moyer 2012). A pictorial rendition of this is shown below (Infographic 2017).

Contrasted with these harms, less than one life per thousand screened would be saved. Considering this, the United States Preventive Services Task Force now recommends against *routine* PSA screening (Moyer 2012).

1,000 men aged 55 to 69 screened every 1 to 4 years for 10 years with a PSA test

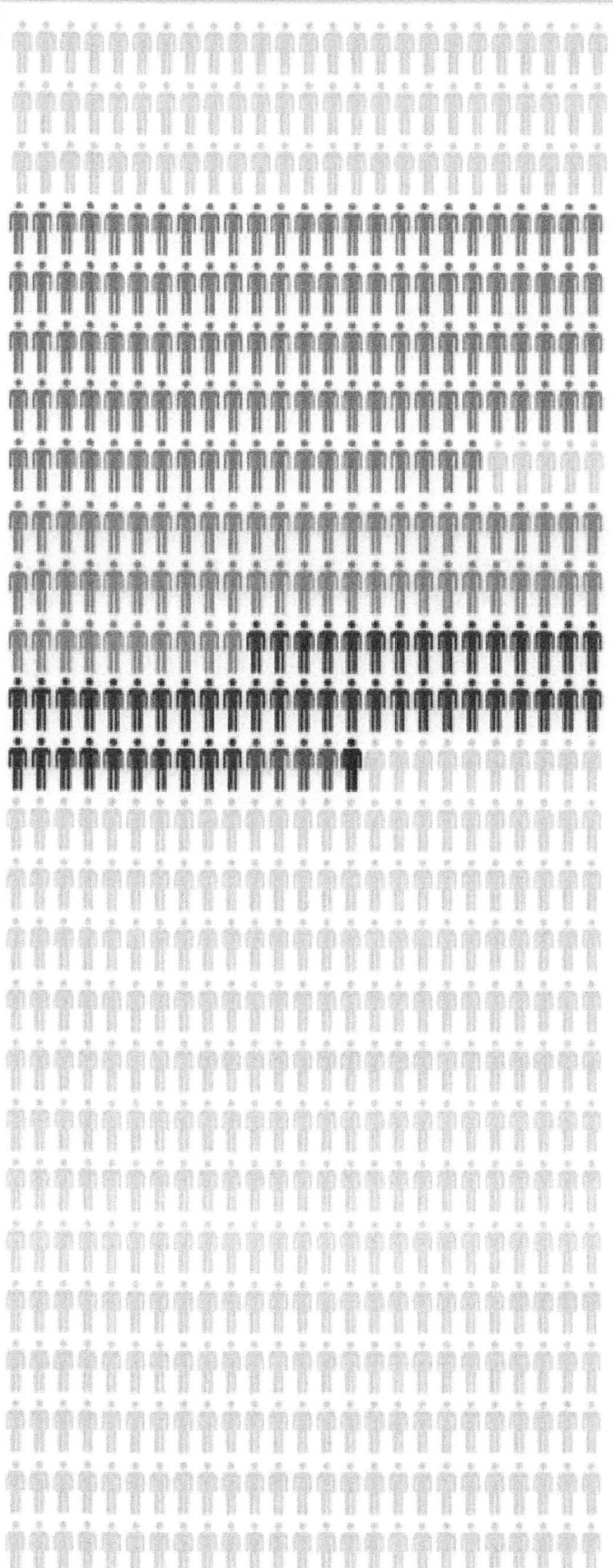

1,000 men screened.

Of these:

100-120

get false-positive results that may cause anxiety and lead to biopsy
(Possible side effects of biopsies include serious infections, pain, and bleeding)

110

get a prostate cancer diagnosis, and of these men:

- at least 50

    will have treatment complications, such as infections, sexual dysfunction, or bladder or bowel control problems

- 4-5

    die from prostate cancer (5 die among men who do not get screened)

- 0-1

    death from prostate cancer is avoided

On the other hand, **though PSA has substantial shortcomings as a *screening* test, it does have value as a *diagnostic* test**. It is useful in follow-up of patients after prostatectomy or radiation therapy. Here a rise in a once depressed PSA level could portend recurrence of prostate cancer. Again, the difference here is that the PSA test is not being applied to the general public, where the false positive rate approximates the true positive rate, but to a population of cancer patients where the possibility of recurrence is high.

Criteria of a Good Screening Test

The World Health Organization (WHO) has developed criteria for evaluating generalized screening tests (Benefits and Risks of Screening Tests 2016). These criteria are self-explanatory:
- Screening should be done only for diseases with serious consequences.
- The test should be reliable and not harmful in itself.
- There must be an effective treatment for the disease when detected at an early stage; and, there must be scientific proof that the treatment is more effective when started before symptoms arise.
- Inconclusive information should be made available to the public, to help people decide whether or not to have the screening test.

An additional requirement is, as indicated above, that the disease should have a significant prevalence in the population being screened. Otherwise, false positives will overwhelm true positives.

The final requirement is that early diagnosis and treatment must lead to an improved health outcome, such as decreased morbidity and mortality, in order to be rationally considered.

Early Diagnosis and Treatment vs. Outcomes

The final requirement, that, in order to be considered, early diagnosis and treatment must improve outcomes, is a requirement not easily met. Consider these examples of cases where early diagnosis does not improve outcomes.

Max Planck Institute Example

The Max Planck Institute for Human Development in Berlin offered this example Illustrating a disconnect between screening and improved outcomes.

Consider two groups of people who all died of cancer at the age of 70, regardless of whether or not they had screening tests. Suppose the group that had screening discovered their cancer at the age of 60 while the group without screening discovered their cancer at the age of 67. Looking only at patients who were alive five years after diagnosis creates the impression that screening prolonged survival. Certainly, all screened patients survived for at least five years and no non-screened patients survived for five years. Nevertheless, all the cancer patients died at the same time. **Early discovery increased awareness time but did not increase survival time** (Benefits and Risks of Screening Tests 2016).

This is shown graphically below (Benefits and Risks of Screening Tests 2016).

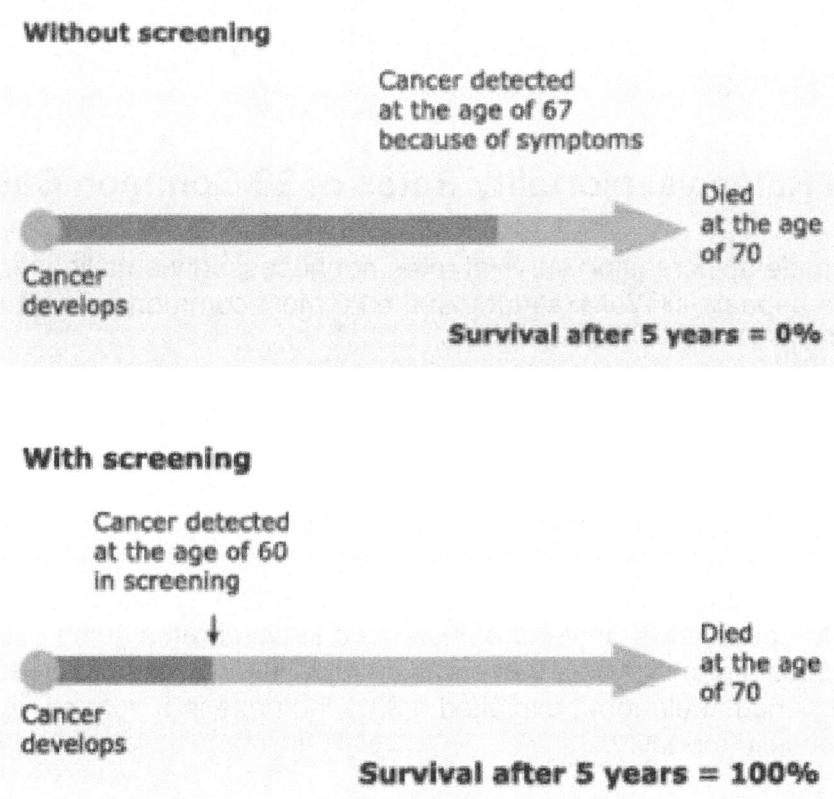

Fig. 22.1 Illustration how screening does not necessarily prolong life, from Benefits and Risks of Screening Tests, 2016.

Mayo Lung Project Example

Another example of early diagnosis from screening not leading to improved outcomes is provided by data from the Mayo Lung Project.

The Mayo Lung Project's subjects consisted of 9211 male smokers randomly assigned to either undergo chest x-ray and sputum cytology every 4 months for 6 years (screening group) or were advised to have the same tests annually (usual care group). The project extended from 1971 to 1983 and the median follow-up period was 20.5 years.

The 5-year survival rate was better in the screened group (35%) than in the usual-care group (19%). In the narrow sub-category of patients with resected early-stage disease, the median survival time was 16.0 years in the screened group versus 5.0 years in the usual-care group. Nevertheless, lung cancer mortality was higher in the screened group (4.4 per 1000 person-years, 95% confidence interval 3.9-4.9) than in the usual-care group (3.9 per 1000 person-years, 95% confidence interval 3.5-4.4) (Marcus 2000).

In summary, **the screened patients did not live longer, they only knew about their disease longer**.

Survival Rates vs. Mortality Rates of 20 Common Cancers

A final example of increasing survival rates not necessarily entailing increased years of life appears in Welch's study of the 20 most common solid cancer types (Welch 2000).

The Welch investigators examined data from the National Cancer Institute's Surveillance, Epidemiology, and End Results (SEER) Program. They noted that from 1950 to 1995 there was an increase in 5-year survival for all of the 20 tumor types, ranging from 3% for pancreatic cancer to 50% for prostate cancer.

However, during that period, mortality rates declined for 12 tumor types but increased for the other 8. Instead of *increased* survival rates being associated with *decreased* mortality rates, there was, in fact, little correlation. Spectacularly, during that period, melanoma exhibited a 39% increase in 5-year survival *and* a 161% *increase* in mortality.

The take-home point here is that increased survival rates do *not* necessarily mean decreased mortality rates.

Lead-Time Bias

The tendency to confuse a longer time from diagnosis until death with a longer time from beginning of the disease until death is called **"lead-time bias."** It **makes survival time seem longer and creates a false impression of the advantages of screenings** and the effectiveness of treatments.

Lead-time bias misleads in another way – it removes some of the subjects from the study. By prolonging the time from diagnosis of a disease until death from that specific disease, it **prolongs the time in which comorbidities can cause death**. If not addressed, this could create the appearance of a subject in the study having had the disease but surviving it. This is another reason to record deaths from any cause, i.e., all-cause mortality, and to include it when drawing conclusions from the study.

Overdiagnosis

Screening may uncover disease instances that progress so slowly as never to become known during the patient's lifetime. This **overdiagnosis inflates the prevalence of the disease**.

Overdiagnosis falsely increases the sensitivity of the test. Intuitively, the test sensitivity that interests us is the sensitivity to identify disease having a clinical outcome, not one so indolent as to be inconsequential. Mathematically, sensitivity is true positives / (true positives + false negatives). Since overdiagnosis inflates the number of true positives, it inflates the sensitivity.

Overdiagnosis skews stage distribution of a malignant disease as it captures a disproportionate number of cases that stay in a lower stage for a longer time (Bajwa 2017). This point is more than academic. It tends to over-represent indolent cases of a disease compared to aggressive cases. But, if the two types are not otherwise distinguishable, a newly diagnosed patient, and his or her physician, want to know the likelihood that this case will behave aggressively, not how many of patients now alive have the indolent vs. the aggressive form.

Overdiagnosis was a factor hypothesized in the Mayo Lung Project for the findings of undiminished mortality despite an increased level of screening (Marcus 2000).

All Cause Mortality

All cause mortality is another indicator of whether screening improves outcomes. All cause mortality can remain the same despite early diagnosis in various circumstances.
- Increased diagnosis leads to increased medical or surgical treatment and patients die from complications of surgery or chemotherapy.
- Patients die from a comorbidity or something else.

In either case, the screening avails the patient little if the patient dies at the same time from another cause.

Hidden Biases in Screening

William Black has raised another issue illuminated by comparison of disease-specific mortality with all-cause mortality. He has suggested that *screening related disease-specific mortality may harbor hidden biases* (Black 2002).

Black examined 12 randomized trials of cancer screening (seven of mammography, three of fecal occult blood detection, and two of chest x-ray screening for lung cancer).

Black subtracted disease-specific mortality in the screened group from that in the control group and did the same for all-cause mortality. When he compared the differences in the two mortality measures, he found that in five of the 12 trials, differences in the two mortality rates went in opposite directions.

Further, in four of these five trials, disease-specific mortality was lower in the screened group than in the control group, whereas all-cause mortality was the same or higher. In two of the remaining seven trials, the mortality rate differences were in the same direction but the difference in all-cause mortality exceeded the disease-specific mortality in the control group.

Black concluded that because all-cause mortality is not affected by bias in classifying cause of death, disparity between all-cause mortality and disease-specific mortality might indicate bias in disease-specific mortality findings. He suggests that biases potentially affecting disease-specific findings are **sticky-diagnosis bias** and **slippery-linkage bias**.

Sticky-diagnosis Bias

Sticky-diagnosis bias is an availability and confirmatory bias that Groopman calls "diagnosis momentum" (Groopman 2010). It **favors the persistence of a diagnosis or avoidance of a diagnosis**.

Sticky-diagnosis bias may have been involved in the excess lung cancer mortality observed in the screened group of the Mayo Lung Project (Marcus 2000). Black cites the potential for deaths from another cause in the screened group being attributed instead to the target cancer because the target cancer had been previously diagnosed in that group. Likewise, he considers that deaths from the target cancer in the control group may be falsely attributed to another cause because the target cancer had *not* been previously diagnosed in the subjects of that group.

Slippery-linkage Bias

Slippery-linkage bias allows the victims of a suspicious screening result that die from the complications of further workup or treatment to escape detection because their deaths are attributed to more proximate causes such as pneumonia, pulmonary embolism, or cardiac event.

Conclusion

The conclusion on screening is short and sweet. Screening is useful only when the screened group exhibits lower death rates as indicated by all cause mortality statistics.

References

Bajwa, A. (n.d.). Lung cancer screening Past, present and the future. Retrieved October 4, 2017, from http://www.bing.com/cr?IG=037E993C940B46AFA9ED6AD16697DCDF&CID=00 C9CA0D47E56462279DC11C46E36553&rd=1&h=-1Bc41ioO5iaJdslew6cAayFZgY7-VZEr8-FKHX0_co&v=1&r=http%3a%2f%2faction.lung.org%2fsite%2fDocServer%2fDr._Bajwa_lung_cancer_screening_grand_rounds.pdf%3fdocID%3d26269&p=DevEx ,5032.1

Benefits and risks of screening tests. (2016, December 27). Retrieved October 04, 2017, from https://www.ncbi.nlm.nih.gov/pubmedhealth/PMH0072602/

Black, W. C., Haggstrom, D. A., & Welch, G. (2002). All-Cause Mortality in Randomized Trials of Cancer Screening. CancerSpectrum Knowledge Environment,94(3), 167-173. doi:10.1093/jnci/94.3.167

Groopman, J. E. (2010). *How doctors think*. Carlton North, Vic.: Scribe Publications.

https://www.cdc.gov/datastatistics/index.html

Infographic: Benefits and Harms of PSA Screening for Prostate Cancer. (2017, June 06). Retrieved October 03, 2017, from https://prevention.cancer.gov/news-and-events/news/infographic-benefits-and

Marcus, P. M., Bergstralh, E. J., Fagerstrom, R. M., Williams, D. E., Fontana, R., Taylor, W. F., & Prorok, P. C. (2000). Lung Cancer Mortality in the Mayo Lung Project: Impact of Extended Follow-up. JNCI Journal of the National Cancer Institute,92(16), 1308-1316. doi:10.1093/jnci/92.16.1308

Moyer, V. A. (2012). Screening for Prostate Cancer: U.S. Preventive Services Task Force Recommendation Statement. Annals of Internal Medicine,157(2), 120. doi:10.7326/0003-4819-157-2-201207170-00459

SEER Cancer Statistics Review 1973-1996. (n.d.). Retrieved December 19, 2017, from https://www.bing.com/cr?IG=FE7001B06E8B4F3D87C3A6A796E65A58&CID=2 735B435223D6260260BBF68239263DE&rd=1&h=IhYkS1rTZ1SLYYQJX8- xZNmMbKSQz_uRxo6PJtq8tBk&v=1&r=https%3a%2f%2fseer.cancer.gov%2farc hive%2fcsr%2f1973_1996%2fappendix.pdf&p=DevEx,5080.1

Welch, H. G. (2000). Are Increasing 5-Year Survival Rates Evidence of Success Against Cancer? *Jama,283*(22), 2975. doi:10.1001/jama.283.22.2975

Further Reading

Groopman, J. E. (2010). *How doctors think*. Carlton North, Vic.: Scribe Publications.

Welch, H. G. (2000). Are Increasing 5-Year Survival Rates Evidence of Success Against Cancer? *Jama,283*(22), 2975. doi:10.1001/jama.283.22.2975

Medical Studies

Chapter 23: Flawed Studies

An avalanche of medical and scientific studies presents itself daily in the print media and online. The studies are often financed by organizations with special interests and are implemented by investigators under immense pressure to publish. These **conditions are strongly conducive to the proliferation of flawed studies**. Here we examine some of the flaws that frequently compromise studies.

Poor Replicability

Critical to the scientific method is replicability. Replicability begins with study design and reporting. Studies lose credibility if they are not reproducibly designed and not reported in sufficient detail that they can be reconstructed independently.

The **requirement of independent replicability is a safeguard that the results obtained in a study are not the consequence of local conditions in the lab or in the population being studied**.

Replicability also helps deal with the problems of statistical uncertainty inherent in an investigation. The level of statistical uncertainty that we traditionally accept is that the probability of rejecting the true results of a study is less than 5%. These odds are good but not perfect. However, they improve each time the study is replicated independently, as 5% of 5% is only 0.25%.

The key is that each of the replications is independent. When the same team performs the replications, the possibility exists that the same systematic errors are introduced at each replication.

A significant example of poor replicability is the famous Mozart Effect study of 1994 by Rauscher's team at UC Irvine. The study concluded, "We have shown that music training can improve the spatial reasoning of three-year-olds" (Rauscher 1994). Nevertheless, the only successful replications were from the original research team. Subsequent studies were unable to detect the effect (Črnčec 2006; McKelvie 2002; Chabris 2012, p. 191).

Non-Random Samples

Next, we consider the problem of sample composition. A reliable sample must accurately reflect the composition of the broader population sampled. This requires that **each individual in the population have an equal chance of being included in the sample**.

When multiple samples are obtained from a population for comparison of drugs or interventions, they must each accurately represent the broader population. First, this allows application of results to the broader population. Second, it assures that the samples accurately represent one another, thus promoting confidence that they are alike in all respects other than the measured variable.

Nevertheless, this representativeness of samples to the broader population and to each other is more difficult to accomplish than is usually assumed.

The editors of the *Literary Digest* obviously felt that nothing could be more representative than a poll. Accordingly, they undertook to predict the results of the presidential election of 1936 between Franklin Roosevelt and Alf Landon from a poll of 10 million people drawn from telephone lists and lists of their subscribers. About 2.5 million of the 10 million responded to the poll. The poll predicted an overwhelming victory for Republican Landon, but Democrat Roosevelt beat Landon in a landslide.

The *Literary Digest* editors failed to consider that their "representative" poll was based on people who had the discretionary income for magazine subscriptions and home phones, at a time when the country was in the grip of a depression. They failed to consider that their subjects had a higher educational level than the general voting population. Finally, they failed to consider the huge number of non-responders in their poll.

One might assume that experimenters and clinicians should do much better than the *Literary Digest* editors in determining representativeness. However, medical professionals are also capable of conscious and unconscious manipulations that render sample selection unrepresentative. The clinician might not enroll certain patients on the assumption that they would not be interested in the study, would not do well, or might drop out. The clinician might bias toward enrolling the most familiar patients for the most familiar treatment and enrolling unfamiliar or more desperate patients for the newer treatment.

The **best way to insure representative samples is to randomize** enrollment into the study. Randomization of enrollment can be accomplished by having each potential subject call a phone number for a computer generated random number (Goldacre 2011, p 51). Other methods might involve giving each subject an envelope with a computer generated random number on a slip inside (Greenhalgh 2014, p. 34).

However, randomness and representativeness in the sample selection is no guarantee of validity of the conclusions if some elements of the sample are not counted or some elements are counted more than once. Unfortunately, both situations easily occur.

Elements Escaping Counting

Some **elements of the sample escape counting when study dropouts are not recorded**. Dropouts are more likely to include study subjects not responding to the drug or intervention as well as study subjects having intolerable side effects. Consequently, removing dropouts biases the outcome of the study in favor of the drug or intervention. Study dropouts must be reported since they influence the degree of confidence that one has in the study.

As mentioned by Shah (Shah, 2011), the comparison of treatment groups that includes all the patients originally allocated after randomization is called **intention-to-treat analysis.** On the other hand, the bias-prone approach that excludes dropouts and includes only those patients who completed the treatment is called **per-protocol analysis.**

An example of an investigation with a high dropout rate is the study of Simpson and Lindenmayer (Simpson 1997). This study compared the extrapyramidal side effects of risperidone versus haloperidol in the treatment of schizophrenic patients. However, this study enrolled 523 schizophrenic patients, of whom only 253 completed the study. The composition of such a large number of dropouts can seriously influence the results of the study.

Elements Counted Multiple Times

While sometimes, as seen above, elements of a sample may escape counting, at other times, **elements of a sample can be counted multiple times**. This occurs **when the same study is published multiple times** under different titles or different authors. More often, portions of the same data are published under different titles by different authors of the same team.

Aside from creating the illusion that the same conclusion is reached in several studies, these multiple publications actually skew the statistical conclusions. This occurs because meta-studies consolidate the data from multiple smaller studies with the goal of producing a more accurate conclusion from a larger database. **When the same data appear as multiple studies, they are counted multiple times and skew the outcome of the meta-study**.

In 1997, Tramer searched reports on ondansetron's effect on postoperative emesis. He found that 17% of published reports and 28% of patient data were duplicated and that none of these reports cross-referenced the original source. He found that data duplication led to an overestimation of ondansetron's antiemetic effect by 23%. Notably, trials reporting greater treatment effects were significantly more likely to be duplicated (Tramer 1997; Gigerenzer 2013, location 1449 of 5166).

Detection of Non-Randomization

Although many studies claim to be randomized, critical thinking entails examination of the method of randomization, how scrupulously the method is executed, and how the data are treated once randomization is complete. The criterion of description is that the study must be described in sufficient detail to permit the reader to repeat the study. Certainly, **if the method of randomization is not fully explained, the results of the study are far less credible**.

Additionally, studies must describe in detail how dropouts from the study are handled. Dropouts from a study are usually the non-responders. **Failure to count the dropouts typically biases the study in favor of the group that had the drug or intervention**.

Inadequate Blinding

A major problem in studies is **expectation bias, in which expectation on the part of subjects or experimenters, patients or physicians, influences the outcome of the study**. When patients expect improvement from a treatment, they report it. When physicians expect to find improvement from a treatment, they find it. This is the basis for the placebo effect and it perpetuates the survival of snake oil treatments.

In 1996, an experiment by Majeed called attention to the pervasiveness of expectation bias. Prior to 1996, several studies had concluded that patients who had had laparoscopic cholecystectomy recovered more quickly than patients who had had open cholecystectomy. Then Majeed did a study in which both patients having had laparoscopic cholecystectomy and patients having had open cholecystectomy left the operating room with identical dressings complete with bloodstains. Neither the patients nor their caregivers knew which surgery the patients had had. The patients having had laparoscopic cholecystectomy were found to have recovered no more quickly than those having had the open surgery. This raised the issue of whether the laparoscopically operated patients were simply discharged sooner because they were expected to recover more quickly (Majeed 1996).

Optimum blinding is **double blinding, in which neither the subjects, nor the experimenters know, *or can determine,* who is in the treatment group and who is in the control group**. Both groups receive the same treatment, attention, and follow-up. These precautions involve expense that can reduce the size of the study. Hence, there may be an incentive to shortcut the precautions.

A big problem in blinding is often experimental design of the treatment intervention. It may be an easy matter to simulate treatment pills with placebos of identical size, color, shape, and weight, dispensed from identical containers;

but, this is more difficult in an investigation of the effectiveness of acupuncture. Here blinding to the intervention might involve sham acupuncture with needles placed in the wrong locations (Goldacre 2011, p. 48). Even so, the practitioner here is not blinded, and neither is any patient familiar with the theory underlying the practice.

Critical thinking about studies requires recognition of the problems posed in the achievement of adequate double blinding. It also requires willingness to suspend judgment or reduce confidence in studies in which inadequate blinding is suspected or in which adequate blinding appears to be unachievable.

Surrogate Outcome Measures

A major problem with outcome measures is the surrogate outcome measure. **In surrogate outcome measures, one parameter is measured as a supposed index of the parameter of true interest**. Sometimes surrogate outcomes are needed for ethical or practical reasons. Other times they replace true outcomes for reasons of convenience or obfuscation.

An example of a legitimate surrogate outcome measure is the initial study of a new drug in animals. This is a surrogate, but a necessary and preliminary one, to testing in humans.

Another necessary surrogate study might be the testing in animals for the long-term effects of a new drug. Here it might be impractical to follow the animals for several years, so instead, the drug being tested might be administered at a dosage several times higher than anticipated in its therapeutic usage.

However, the fact remains that surrogate outcome measures are not measures of the parameter of true interest. This reduces confidence in conclusions from them and must be considered in critically evaluating studies.

Statistical vs. Clinical Significance

Statistical significance is, well, statistical. However, clinical significance is practical.

There can be a **high degree of certainty that one drug is minimally more effective than another** in a large, well-constructed trial. However, the minimal superiority of the new drug may not offer a significant advantage to the patient. To make matters worse, its minimal advantage in primary effect may be far outweighed by its side effects.

This is one reason not to do some screening tests. Those tests may secure only minimal benefit but lead to many false positives, so many false positives that more patients would be injured in investigations and therapies in investigation of the false positives than would be injured by missing a few results by not doing screening.

It is important in the critical evaluation of studies that claims of significance be distinguished: mathematical from medical, statistical from practical.

Compromised Meta-Analyses

The major advantage of the **meta-study** is that it **combines the samples from many smaller studies into a larger sample that should conduce to a more reliable conclusion**.

However, meta-analyses are themselves subject to compromise.

First, in order to combine the samples from many smaller studies, the smaller studies must have comparable protocols, definitions of terms, control conditions, participants, and outcome measures (Gigerenzer 2013, location 2118 of 5166). Few meta-analyses meet all of these criteria and an attempt to force-fit them compromises the credibility of the meta-analysis.

Second, the meta-analysis propagates the publication bias that affected its component primary studies.

Third, as indicated above in Tramer's ondansetron study, the meta-analysis is sensitive to errors occasioned by multiple publications of its component studies or component data ((Tramer 1997; Gigerenzer 2013, location 1449 of 5166).

These failings may not be trivial. A 1997 study published in the New England Journal of Medicine (*NEJM*) compared published meta-analyses with subsequent large well-designed trials and found that the meta-analyses failed to predict the outcome of the later well-designed trials 35% of the time (Novella 2013, Kindle location 3777 of 16057).

The take-home point is that critical thinking about studies requires that **even meta-analyses be checked against large, well-constructed, random controlled trials.**

Sharpshooter Revisited

Earlier we conjured the image of a man haphazardly shooting at the side of a barn. After producing a random array of bullet holes on the barn side, he strides up to the barn, selects one of the bullet holes (or, better, an area where a few bullet holes are clustered), draws a bull's eye around this, and proclaims that the bull's eye attests to the accuracy of his shooting.

Surprisingly, this phenomenon can be applied to impose significance upon the random data acquired in studies. Goldacre (Goldacre 2014) references a study by Jureidini examining the infamous "Study 329," the data from which became available only as the result of the litigation *Beverly Smith vs. SmithKline Beecham*.

Study 329, in its original protocols, specified the examination of paroxetine vs. placebo according to two primary outcomes and six secondary ones. At the end of the trial, there was no significant difference between paroxetine and placebo for any of these outcomes. However, at least 19 more outcomes were also measured. Of these, four gave a positive result for paroxetine and these were reported as if they were the main outcomes (Jureidini 2008).

The **reason that outcomes other than the originally specified ones should not be repurposed and reported as main outcomes is that they may not have been controlled for in designing the original experiment**. Consequently, if these incidental outcomes suggest a potential hypothesis, that hypothesis must be clearly specified and a dedicated experiment, controlled for likely confounding variables, must be designed to test it. This is the reason for clearly specifying the tested hypothesis at the outset. As Goldacre writes, **"You cannot find your hypothesis in your results"** (Goldacre 2011, Kindle Locations 2837-2852).

Underpowered Studies and Their Detection

The purpose of a study is to draw a conclusion about a larger population from the examination of a smaller sample population.

Consider the example of a new drug, which in a preliminary study on 20 subjects with an average systolic blood pressure of 140 mmHg, seems to lower systolic blood pressure to an average of 125 mmHg. We wish to know how this will behave in a larger population, say of 10,000,000 people.

Further, we realize that systolic blood pressure lowering from 140 mmHg to 125 mmHg is a mean that holds even if many subjects show no effect and many show a systolic lowering to 110 mmHg. However, a drop in systolic pressure to 110 mmHg might create symptoms in some patients, and a 0 mmHg reduction would be useless.

Consequently, we wish to be 95% sure that systolic blood pressure reduction will be to the average of 125 mmHg and be in the range 120 -130 mmHg. In other words, we desire a probability of 0.95 in an average of 125 mmHg with a confidence interval of +/- 5 mmHg (p = 0.95, CI +/- 5 mmHg). How large a sample do we need to investigate in order to have this confidence?

Fortunately, there exist formulas (Finding Sample Size for Estimating a Population Proportion, n. d.) and internet calculator tools that enable this determination. One of these calculator tools is http://www.macorr.com/sample-size-calculator.htm (Market Research Survey Company, n. d.) and another is https://www.surveysystem.com/sscalc.htm (Survey Software, n. d.). The aforementioned formula and tools are basic and without sophistication, but they do provide a starting point.

Using either of these tools, we can plug in the values of 95% for confidence level and 10,000,000 for population. The tools require that we enter the confidence interval as a percent. Since we desire a confidence interval of 10 mmHg at a baseline of 140 mmHg, the confidence interval expressed in percent is 10/140 or 7%. On entering 7% and pressing the "calculate" button, either tool yields a sample size of 196 subjects.

The conclusion is that if the sample studied contains at least 196 subjects, and it shows the new drug to be associated with a reduction of average systolic blood pressure from 140 mmHg to 125 mmHg with a confidence interval of 120-130 mmHg, then we can be 95% sure that this applies to a population of 10,000,000,

However, this is so only if the sample studied is at least 196 subjects. If the study contains less than 196 subjects, then it is too small to justify this conclusion and the study is said to be *underpowered.*

In sum, having formulas and tools for calculation of appropriate sample size is immensely beneficial in critically evaluating medical and scientific studies. With them, **it is possible, on reading a study, to infer whether or not the sample size is large enough to support the conclusions of the study**.

Conclusion

"Studies show." These are two words that should immediately switch on all of our critical thinking circuits. Studies can be flawed in many ways, including non-replicability, skewed samples, missing or repeated data, inadequate blinding, surrogate outcome measures, confusion between statistical and clinical significance, under powering, and results-generated hypotheses. Conclusions cannot compel assent based solely on the fact that they have data attached and have penetrated the, sometimes porous, barrier into publication.

References

Chabris, C. F., & Simons, D. J. (2012). *The invisible gorilla: and other ways our intuitions deceive us*. New York: MJF Books.

Cognitive bias. (2017, April 09). Retrieved April 11, 2017, from https://en.wikipedia.org/wiki/Cognitive_bias

Črnčec, R., Wilson, S. J., & Prior, M. (2006). No Evidence for the Mozart Effect in Children. Music Perception,23(4), 305-318. doi:10.1525/mp.2006.23.4.305

Gigerenzer, G. (2013). Better doctors, better patients, better decisions: envisioning health care 2020;. Cambridge, Mass.: MIT Press.

Goldacre, B. (2014). Bad pharma: how drug companies mislead doctors and harm patients. New York: Faber & Faber, Inc., an affiliate of Farrar, Straus and Giroux.

Goldacre, B. (2011). Bad science: quacks, hacks, and big pharma flacks. Toronto: Emblem Editions.

Greenhalgh, T. (2014). *How to Read a Paper: The Basics of Evidence-based Medicine*. Wiley-Blackwell.

Jureidini, J. N. (2008). Clinical trials and drug promotion: Selective reporting of study 329 . International Journal of Risk and Safety in Medicine,20, 73-81. doi:10.3233/JRS-2008-0426

Majeed, A., Troy, G., Smythe, A., Reed, M., Stoddard, C., Peacock, J., . . . Nicholl, J. (1996). Randomised, prospective, single-blind comparison of laparoscopic versus small-incision cholecystectomy. The Lancet,347(9007), 989-994. doi:10.1016/s0140-6736(96)90143-9

Market research survey company | MaCorr Research. (n.d.). Retrieved July 30, 2017, from http://www.macorr.com/sample-size-calculator

McKelvie, P., & Low, J. (2002). Listening to Mozart does not improve children's spatial ability: Final curtains for the Mozart effect. British Journal of Developmental Psychology,20(2), 241-258. doi:10.1348/026151002166433

Novella, S., Gorski, D., & Crislip, M. (2013). Science-Based Medicine: Guide to Critical Thinking. Fort Lauderdale, FL: James Randi Educational Foundation. Kindle Edition.

Psychopharmacology,17(3), 194-201. doi:10.1097/00004714-199706000-00010

Reisin, E. (july 1, 1997). Lisinopril Versus Hydrochlorothiazide in Obese Hypertensive Patients. *Hypertension*.

Shah, P. B. (2011). Intention-to-treat and per-protocol analysis. *Canadian Medical Association Journal,183*(6), 696-696. doi:10.1503/cmaj.111-2033

Simpson, G. M., & Lindenmayer, J. (1997). Extrapyramidal Symptoms in Patients Treated With Risperidone. Journal of Clinical

Survey Software - The Survey System. (n.d.). Retrieved July 30, 2017, from http://www.surveysystem.com/sscalc

Tramer, M. R., Reynolds, D. J., Moore, R. A., & Mcquay, H. J. (1997). Impact of covert duplicate publication on meta-analysis: a case study. Bmj,315(7109), 635-640. doi:10.1136/bmj.315.7109.635

Further Reading

Chabris, C. F., & Simons, D. J. (2012). *The invisible gorilla: and other ways our intuitions deceive us*. New York: MJF Books.

Gigerenzer, G. (2013). Better doctors, better patients, better decisions: envisioning health care 2020;. Cambridge, Mass.: MIT Press.

Goldacre, B. (2014). Bad pharma: how drug companies mislead doctors and harm patients. New York: Faber & Faber, Inc., an affiliate of Farrar, Straus and Giroux.

Goldacre, B. (2011). Bad science: quacks, hacks, and big pharma flacks. Toronto: Emblem Editions.

Greenhalgh, T. (2014). *How to Read a Paper: The Basics of Evidence-based Medicine*. Wiley-Blackwell.

Novella, S., Gorski, D., & Crislip, M. (2013). Science-Based Medicine: Guide to Critical Thinking. Fort Lauderdale, FL: James Randi Educational Foundation. Kindle Edition.

Tramer, M. R., Reynolds, D. J., Moore, R. A., & Mcquay, H. J. (1997). Impact of covert duplicate publication on meta-analysis: a case study. Bmj,315(7109), 635-640. doi:10.1136/bmj.315.7109.635

Chapter 24: Fraudulent Studies

We are repulsed by the thought that there might be cases of outright fraud in scientific and medical research. Nevertheless, and possibly, because this is unthinkable, it has frequently gone undetected for long periods. However, the fact is that fraud exists and it alerts us to the need of critical evaluation of medical and scientific studies.

Fraud -- Fabrication and Falsification

The US Public Health Service defines **fabrication** as **"making up data or results and recording or reporting them."** It defines **falsification** as **"changing or omitting data or results such that the research is not accurately represented"** (Department of Health and Human Services 2005, Title 42: Section 93.103).

Fang Study

Fang and colleagues, in 2012, published a study of the **2,047 articles listed as retracted by PubMed up until May 3, 2012**. The study found **that fraud or suspected fraud involved 43.4% of the retractions**. Following fraud, error accounted for 21.3% of the retractions. Plagiarism or duplicate publication involved many of the remaining retractions.

Fang's study also found that 17 authors had 10 or more retractions, with fraud being the cause in the cases of all authors except one. One author had 80 retractions, one had 36, and one had 21 (Fang 2012, Table S2).

The Fang study found that in 119 retractions, the journal provided no reason for the action. In many other retractions, the authors of the original article wrote the retraction, which proved to be "uninformative or opaque."

The investigators concluded, "Our findings underscore the importance of vigilance by reviewers, editors, and readers" (Fang 2012).

Yoshitaka Fujii Case

Yoshitaka Fujii is a Japanese anesthesiologist widely published over many years, especially for his investigations of granisetron for postoperative nausea and vomiting. In 2012, UK anesthesiologist J. Carlisle published in *Anaesthesia* an exhaustive analysis of distribution of variables from 168 clinical trials published by Fujii over 20 years. Carlisle was concerned that the frequency distributions were much less variable than expected by chance (Carlisle 2012).

These findings prompted an investigation of 212 Fujii papers by the Japanese Society of Anesthesiologists. **Of the 212 papers, 172 were found fraudulent, of which 126 were found "totally fabricated"** (George 2015).

Harry Snyder Case

In 1994, Harry Snyder was a dermatologist and scientist at BioCryst Pharmaceuticals of Birmingham, Alabama, a company in which Snyder had substantial financial interest. Snyder was testing BCX-34 to be used as a topical ointment in the treatment of psoriasis and cutaneous T-cell lymphoma. In February 1995, a BioCryst press release claimed highly favorable results for BCX-34, especially for cutaneous T-cell lymphoma.

However, a retraction of the press release appeared in June 1995 with the notation of "no statistically significant drug effect." Audits by the company and the FDA resulted in charges of falsification of data. Snyder received a felony conviction and was sentenced to three years in prison (George 2015).

Detecting Fraud

At first, it seems impossible to protect oneself from falling victim to fraudulent research studies. Certainly, fraudulent cases as the above typically come to attention through sophisticated statistical analysis such as Carlisle's or through whistleblower tips. These methods are unavailable to the casual reader of the technical literature.

However, the following circumstances can raise suspicion.
- A **large amount of studies from one person**, especially if that person does not have access to a large team of co-investigators.
- A **study with results widely disparate from other studies** of the same hypothesis.
- A **study whose results strongly support an agenda of the organization financing the study**.

Fortunately, however, resources such as the following are available to investigate the backgrounds of study authors
- **RetractionWatch.com** is a respected site that follows retractions and has a search function to check authors for retractions. It is important for two reasons. First, retractions of studies are frequently overlooked and the studies continue to be cited. Second, authors with multiple retractions legitimately lose credibility as investigators.

- **www.ori.hhs.gov** is the web site of the Office of Research Integrity in the US Department of Health and Human Services. The site has a Bulletin Board of Administrative Actions, a library of Misconduct Case Summaries, and a search function for locating authors.

A check of these resources is an investment in good information.

References

Carlisle, J. B. (2012). The analysis of 168 randomised controlled trials to test data integrity. Anaesthesia,67(5), 521-537. doi:10.1111/j.1365-2044.2012.07128.x

Department of Health and Human Services - ORI. (2005, May 17). Retrieved July 12, 2017, from https://www.bing.com/cr?IG=7F2A26B7CA6048BE8A0FE9718DB52171&CID=0 9D7C2E08ECC62123EE7C85D8FCA6394&rd=1&h=ik3ooSl41xD7kJh0hmxUoN XbU4x2d5qTfptqbGX24ms&v=1&r=https%3a%2f%2fori.hhs.gov%2fsites%2fdefa ult%2ffiles%2f42_cfr_parts_50_and_93_2005.pdf&p=DevEx,5061.1

Fang, F. C., Steen, R. G., & Casadevall, A. (2012). Misconduct accounts for the majority of retracted scientific publications. Proceedings of the National Academy of Sciences,109(42), 17028-17033. doi:10.1073/pnas.1212247109

George, S. L., & Buyse, M. (2015). Data fraud in clinical trials. Clinical Investigation,5(2), 161-173. doi:10.4155/cli.14.116

Further Reading

Fang, F. C., Steen, R. G., & Casadevall, A. (2012). Misconduct accounts for the majority of retracted scientific publications. Proceedings of the National Academy of Sciences,109(42), 17028-17033. doi:10.1073/pnas.1212247109

Chapter 25: Publication Bias

Will Rogers famously quipped, "All I know is what I read in the papers, and that's an alibi for my ignorance." Will's comment should be a caution against uncritically absorbing, repeating, and implementing everything seen in print.

Publication Bias Definition

Publication bias is the tendency for the outcome of a study to influence whether or not it is published or disseminated. Specifically, a tendency exists for studies concluding positively to receive more publication than studies indicating "no difference."

Emerson Study – Publication Bias

Emerson and colleagues, in 2010, submitted two versions of a fabricated randomized controlled trial to 238 reviewers in orthopedics journals. The two versions were identical in all respects except that the findings in one were positive and the findings in the other revealed no difference.

Of the 238 invited reviewers, 210 responded and found more errors in the no-difference version. Additionally, they assigned lower methods scores to the no-difference version. Most importantly, 80.0 % of the reviewers recommended publication for the no-difference version while 97.3% recommended publication for the positive version (Emerson 2010).

Dickersin Study – Publication Bias

In 1987, Dickersin and colleagues released a study in which they asked 318 authors of published randomized clinical trials (RCTs) if they had participated in any unpublished RCTs. 156 responded and reported 271 unpublished and 1041 published trials. Of 178 completed *unpublished* RCTs with a trend specified, 26 (14%) favored the new therapy compared to 423 of 767 (55%) favoring the new therapy in *published* reports ($p < 0.001$) (Dickersin 1987).

Easterbrook Study – Publication Bias

In 1991, Easterbrook and colleagues released in *Lancet* a review of 285 studies, 52% of which had been published. The review indicated that studies with statistically significant results were more likely to be published than studies finding no difference between the study groups, with an odds ratio of 2.32 to 1 and a 0.95 confidence interval of 1.25-4.28 (Easterbrook 1991).

Turner Study – Publication Bias

Turner and colleagues released in the *New England Journal of Medicine* in 2008 a study of 12 antidepressants. They obtained from the Food and Drug Administration the total studies of the 12 antidepressants involving 12,564 patients and compared those outcomes with the subset published in the literature.

According to the published literature, 94% of the trials were positive. By contrast, in the total data considered by the FDA, 51% were positive (Turner 2008).

Reasons for Publication Bias

Publication bias may be generated by multiple factors:
- Editors may not be inclined to publish no-difference studies because they are less interesting to readers and may impact advertising.
- Corporate sponsors of the studies may decline to submit for publication studies showing no difference between their own product and placebo.
- Investigators may decline to submit no-difference studies for publication feeling that submitting a no-difference result takes time, is less likely to be published, and does not enhance, or may harm, their academic stature.
- Investigators may not submit studies with disparate conclusions from previously published studies because they fear the inconsistency reflects a shortcoming of their own work.
- Investigators may feel that failing to reject the null hypothesis only formalizes a result of which the scientific community was already aware as the default position.

Detecting Publication Bias

Light and Pillemer in 1984 devised a **simple test for the detection of publication bias** (Light 1984). They reasoned that statistics predicts that in a collection of studies, all with the same independent and dependent variable, the average values of the dependent variable in the studies, i.e., the effect, would be widely distributed around the mean when the populations studied were small. However, when the populations studied were large, the average values of the dependent variable would be more tightly clustered about the mean.

Consequently, if the values of the dependent variable were represented on the x-axis and the population size studied were represented on the y-axis, the **points representing the intersection of sample size and value mean would disperse in the shape of a triangle or upside-down funnel** (See Fig 25.1).

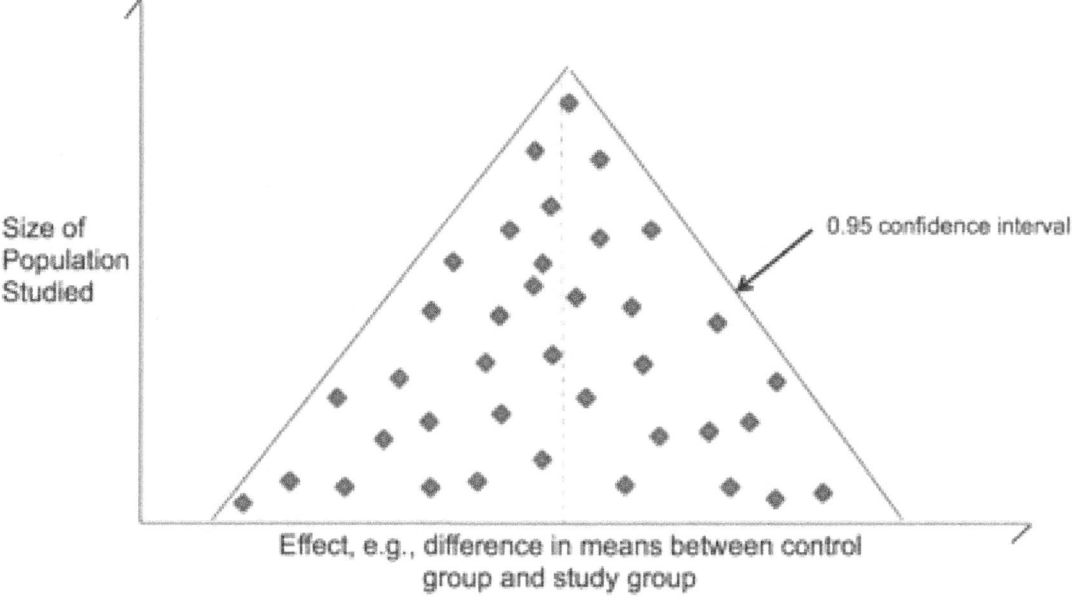

Figure 25.1 Funnel plot not influenced by publication bias.

If the intersection points fail to distribute in such a shape, it suggests that some of the data points are missing (See Figure 25.2).

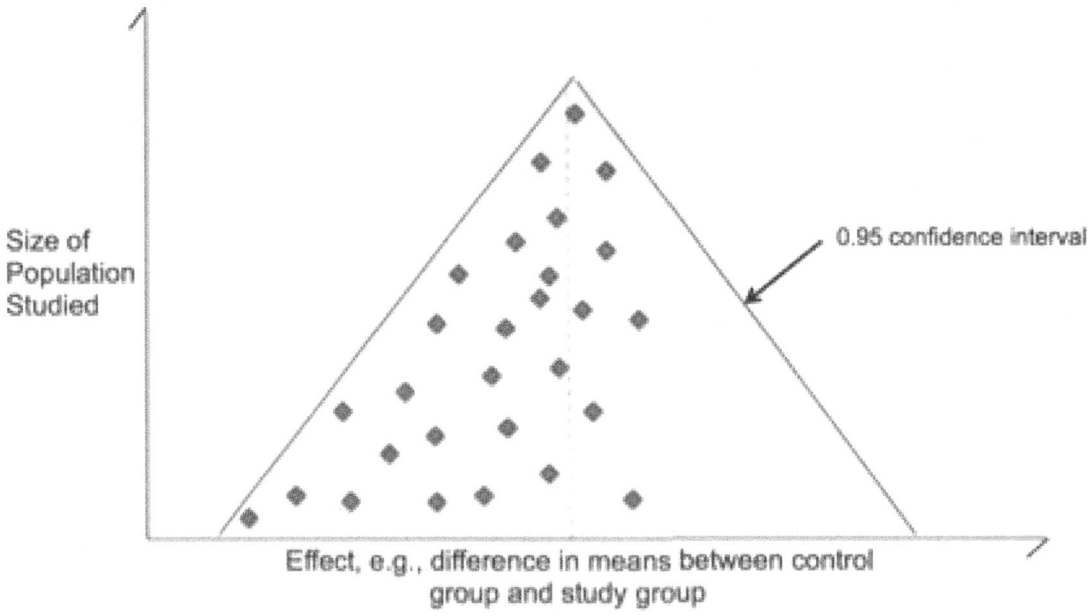

Figure 25.2 Funnel plot influenced by publication bias.

Impact of Publication Bias

Neither the integrity of science nor the legitimate expectations of patients is served when the professional literature is slanted toward positive findings.

The effects of publication bias are negative and far-reaching.
- The bias may not do enough to discourage studies with small populations, which are more likely to report unreliable extreme results.
- The bias may provide inferior data for meta-studies whose compromised conclusions are more likely to influence clinical practice.
- Over-weighted positive results in meta-studies may discourage investigators with no-difference results from submitting their findings for publication.

Possible Countermeasures to Publication Bias

In 1979, Rosenthal first described the problem of publication bias (Rosenthal 1979). Since then, the problem has persisted with little progress.

Some proposals for addressing publication bias are as follows:

- Encourage meta-analyses to search rigorously for both published and unpublished studies (Ahmed 2012).
- Extend to all human trials the present system for FDA drug trials which preregisters all trials involving human subjects in a central database, where they would be accessible to researchers, whether published or not (Novella 2008).
- Encourage researchers to submit negative studies for publication, and encourage journal editors to publish negative results, and not favor positive results that are more likely to grab headlines (Novella 2008).
- Support the public or charitable funding of electronic journals for no-difference results in various research fields (Joober 2012).
- When publishing a clinical trial, provide patient-level data to researchers with dissenting points of view and allow them a brief comment following the article (Lacasse 2013).
- Create high-status publication outlets for studies showing no-difference results (Franco 2014).
- Allocate resources for replication of published studies that are unrepresentative (Franco 2014).

Conclusion

Publication bias is insidious in that it is difficult to know the unseen information. It distorts the information that is seen in the primary studies as well as the overall conclusions in the meta-studies. Finally, it suppresses the conflicting information. Further countermeasures need to be developed and existing countermeasures need to be rigorously implemented.

References

Ahmed, I., Sutton, A. J., & Riley, R. D. (2012). Assessment of publication bias, selection bias, and unavailable data in meta-analyses using individual participant data: a database survey. British Medical Journal,344(Jan03 1), D7762-D7762. doi:10.1136/bmj.d7762

Dickersin, K., Chan, S., Chalmersx, T., Sacks, H., & Smith, H. (1987). Publication bias and clinical trials. Controlled Clinical Trials,8(4), 343-353. doi:10.1016/0197-2456(87)90155-3

Easterbrook, P., Gopalan, R., Berlin, J., & Matthews, D. (1991). Publication bias in clinical research. The Lancet,337(8746), 867-872. doi:10.1016/0140-6736(91)90201-y

Emerson, G. B., Warme, W. J., Wolf, F. M., Heckman, J. D., Brand, R. A., & Leopold, S. S. (2010). Testing for the Presence of Positive-

Franco, A., Malhotra, N., & Simonovits, G. (2014). Publication bias in the social sciences: Unlocking the file drawer. Science,345(6203), 1502-1505. doi:10.1126/science.1255484

Influence on Apparent Efficacy. New England Journal of Medicine,358(3), 252-260. doi:10.1056/nejmsa065779

Ioannidis, J. P. (2005, August). Why Most Published Research Findings Are False. Retrieved June 27, 2017, from https://www.ncbi.nlm.nih.gov/pmc/articles/PMC1182327/

Joober, R., Schmitz, N., Annable, L., & Boksa, P. (2012). Publication bias: What are the challenges and can they be overcome? Journal of Psychiatry & Neuroscience,37(3), 149-152. doi:10.1503/jpn.120065

Lacasse, J. (2013, July 06). Saving Science: It's Time to Solve Publication Bias. Retrieved June 27, 2017, from https://www.madinamerica.com/author/jlacasse/

Leopold, S. S. (2010). Testing for the Presence of Positive-Outcome Bias in Peer Review

Light, R., & Pillemer, D. (1984). . Light RJ, Pillemer DB. Summing Up: The Science of Reviewing Research. Cambridge: Harvard University Press; 1984.Cambridge, MA: Harvard University Press.

Novella, S. (2008, March 11). Do Antidepressants Work? The Effect of Publication Bias. Retrieved June 26, 2017, from https://sciencebasedmedicine.org/do-antidepressants-work-the-effect-of-publication-bias/

Outcome Bias in Peer Review. Archives of Internal Medicine,170(21). doi:10.1001/archinternmed.2010.406

Rosenthal, R. (1979). The file drawer problem and tolerance for null results. Psychological Bulletin,86(3), 638-641. doi:10.1037/0033-2909.86.3.638

Song, F., Hooper, L., & Loke, Y. (2013). Publication bias: what is it? How do we measure it? How do we avoid it? Open Access Journal of Clinical Trials,71-81. doi:10.2147/oajct.s34419

Turner, E. H., Matthews, A. M., Linardatos, E., Tell, R. A., & Rosenthal, R. (2008). Selective Publication of Antidepressant Trials and Its Influence on Apparent Efficacy

Chapter 26: Unpublished Studies

Unpublished studies are a major problem in the overall evaluation of evidence. Certainly, valid conclusions are difficult to draw when only some of the information is available for consideration.

ClinicalTrials.gov

The 1997 FDA Modernization Act attempted to address this issue by creating the website **ClinicalTrials.gov**, which went online in 2000. The Modernization Act required registration of trials for any new drug intended for a serious or life-threatening disease (Goldacre 2014, p. 49).

Then, in 2007, the FDA Amendment Act required registration of all trials of any drug or device involving a site in the US or an application to bring a new drug to market. The **Amendment Act also required posting, within one year of completion, to ClinicalTrials.gov, of summary tables for any trial completed after 2007 on any marketed drug** (Goldacre 2014, p. 52).

Still, however, a study in the *British Medical Journal* by Prayle revealed that **only 22% of trials completed between January 1, 2009 and December 31, 2009 were posted on the site**, although posting was required (Prayle 2012).

Gøtzsche Study and its Aftermath

In 2006, Gøtzsche published a study in the *Journal of the American Medical Association* (*JAMA*) (Gøtzsche 2006) and, two months later, in the *Journal of the Danish Medical Association*. In this study, Gøtzsche and his associates examined the protocols of 44 industry-initiated trials from 1994-1995.

The Gøtzsche group found that in 16 of the trials, the trial sponsor could access the data as it was still accumulating. In 16 more trials, the industrial sponsor could stop the trial at any time for any reason. Further, in only one of these cases did the final report disclose this control by the sponsor over the trial protocol.

Moreover, **in 22 of the 44 trials, the trial protocols stated that the trial sponsor either owned the data or needed to approve the publication manuscript**. This condition was not stated in any of the final trial reports.

The Gøtzsche group had similar findings from a 2004 study of 44 additional trial protocols.

As a consequence of their publication of these findings, the Gøtzsche group became the target of attacks by Lif (Lægemiddelindustriforeningen), the Danish pharmaceutical industry association, as documented in the *British Medical Journal (BMJ)* (Gornall 2009).

The *BMJ* reported that in April 2007, Lif wrote the first of three letters to the Danish Committees on Scientific Dishonesty to accuse the researchers of scientific misconduct. Lif copied some of the letters to the hospital where four of the Gøtzsche group worked, to the Central Scientific-Ethics Committee, to the Danish Medical Association, to the Danish Drug Agency, to the Ministry of Health, to the Ministry of Science, and to the Journal of the Danish Medical Association. About a year after the first accusation, the Committees on Scientific Dishonesty dismissed the charges. Gøtzsche and his group were vindicated.

Goldacre's Countermeasures to Unpublished Studies

Ben Goldacre has offered several countermeasures to the problem of unpublished studies (Goldacre 2014). These are just a few:
- All trials should be registered before they begin.
- All trial results should be published within a year of completion.
- Trial registers such as ClinicalTrials.gov should be used fully.
- Open-access journals such as *Trials* should be used fully. These journals are free to access, have an editorial policy that they will accept any trial report, regardless of result, and solicit negative findings.
- Gagging clauses should be illegal. Such clauses restrict the rights of researchers to publish, discuss, or analyze data from the trials they have conducted, without permission from the funder of the trial.

AllTrials is an international initiative with the mission "All trials registered ... All Trials Reported." The initiative was founded by Ben Goldacre, the *British Medical Journal*, the Center for Evidence-based Medicine, the Cochrane Collaboration, the James Lind Initiative, the Public Library of Science, Sense about Science USA, Dartmouth's Geisel School of Medicine, and the Dartmouth Institute for Health Policy and Clinical Practice.

Conclusion

Finding unpublished studies is a daunting challenge unless one can identify studies initiated and compare them to studies showing published results. *AllTrials* endeavors to do just that. *AllTrials* is a worthy initiative deserving the full support of the medical and scientific communities.

References

Goldacre, B. (2014). Bad pharma: how drug companies mislead doctors and harm patients. New York: Faber & Faber, Inc., an affiliate of Farrar, Straus and Giroux.

Goldacre, B., British Medical Journal, Center for Evidence-based Medicine, Cochrane Collaboration, James Lind Initiative, Public Library of Science, . . . Dartmouth Institute for Health Policy and Clinical Practice. (n.d.). All Trials Registered. All Results Reported. Retrieved August 31, 2017, from http://www.alltrials.net/

Gornall, J. (2009). Industry attack on academics. Bmj,338(Mar09 1). doi:10.1136/bmj.b736

Gøtzsche, P. C., Hróbjartsson, A., Johansen, H. K., Haahr, M. T., Altman, D. G., & Chan, A. (2006). Constraints on Publication Rights in Industry-Initiated Clinical Trials. Jama,295(14), 1641. doi:10.1001/jama.295.14.1645

Prayle, A. P., Hurley, M. N., & Smyth, A. R. (2012). Compliance with mandatory reporting of clinical trial results on ClinicalTrials.gov: cross sectional study. Bmj,344(Jan03 1), D7373-D7373. doi:10.1136/bmj.d7373

Further Reading

Goldacre, B. (2014). Bad pharma: how drug companies mislead doctors and harm patients. New York: Faber & Faber, Inc., an affiliate of Farrar, Straus and Giroux.

Chapter 27: Countermeasures to Misleading Studies

In addition to the aforementioned, there are further countermeasures that we can implement individually, in daily situations, to reduce the impact of misleading studies.

Healthy Skepticism of Industry-Sponsored Studies

Medical care is heavily involved with industry, including the pharmaceutical industry, the medical device industry, and the health care delivery industry. Industry conducts or funds a vast number of studies of its own products.

It comes as no surprise that industry can influence studies in three ways: by biasing the topics studied, biasing the design of clinical trials, and biasing the reporting of results in journals (Gigerenzer 2013, location 171 of 5166).

First, **industry has immense bias toward reporting favorable studies on its products, especially its most profitable products**, such as antihypertensive or antihyperlipidemic medications that patients purchase repeatedly for the rest of their lives.

Second, **investigators are highly biased toward reporting results favorable to the industry when the industry employs or contracts them to study its products**.

Third, many **journals depend heavily on advertising revenue and also publish studies investigating the products of their advertisers**. This introduces a bias toward publishing the favorable studies in preference to the unfavorable studies.

It would be remiss not to consider these influences and to rely solely on the image of the product, the investigators, or the journal in evaluating the credibility of the study.

Systematic Reviews (Cochrane Collaboration)

Another useful countermeasure to being deceived by misleading study conclusions is to consult systematic reviews. **Systematic reviews are examinations of all the available literature according to a predetermined**

search strategy, with predetermined parameters for the data of the study and the quality of the study.

Systematic reviews are time-consuming and difficult to execute but promise to be more immune to bias and error than most studies. The most prominent source of systematic reviews is from Cochrane.org, which uses volunteer evaluators following a rigorous prescribed format to evaluate the literature.

Cochrane reviews are published by John Wiley and Sons. While the abstracts and plain language summary are available free of charge, the entire review may require a subscription. The subscription is provided free of charge by the governments of some foreign countries and the State of Wyoming.

Forest Plot or "Blobbogram"

A **forest plot is a graphical representation of a meta-analysis** (Gurusamy 2017). In turn, a meta-analysis is a study that combines the samples from many smaller studies into a larger sample that should conduce to a more reliable conclusion.

The forest plot makes the meta-analysis easier to understand. The plot first appeared in the 1980s and reached its present form in the 1990s. Cochrane Reviews (Cochrane.org) makes extensive use of forest plots and has adopted a stylized forest plot as its logo.

The forest plot below is from K. Gurusamy (Gurusamy 2017) and summarizes six studies.

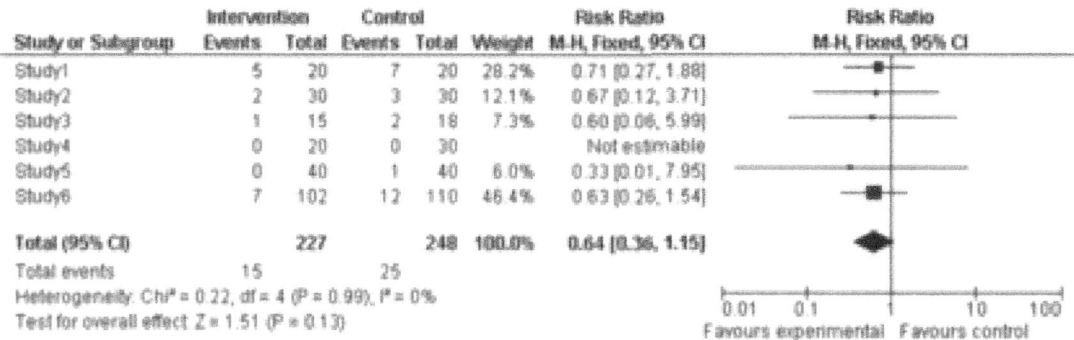

Study or Subgroup	Intervention Events	Total	Control Events	Total	Weight	Risk Ratio M-H, Fixed, 95% CI	Risk Ratio M-H, Fixed, 95% CI
Study1	5	20	7	20	28.2%	0.71 [0.27, 1.88]	
Study2	2	30	3	30	12.1%	0.67 [0.12, 3.71]	
Study3	1	15	2	18	7.3%	0.60 [0.06, 5.99]	
Study4	0	20	0	30		Not estimable	
Study5	0	40	1	40	6.0%	0.33 [0.01, 7.95]	
Study6	7	102	12	110	46.4%	0.63 [0.26, 1.54]	
Total (95% CI)		227		248	100.0%	0.64 [0.36, 1.15]	
Total events	15		25				

Heterogeneity: Chi² = 0.22, df = 4 (P = 0.99), I² = 0%
Test for overall effect: Z = 1.51 (P = 0.13)

0.01 0.1 1 10 100
Favours experimental Favours control

Figure 27.1 Gurusamy, K. (2017, September 14). Interpretation of Forest Plots -
Part 1. Lecture presented at Interpretation of Forest Plots - Part 1, London, UK.
Lecture - University College London

The lengths of the horizontal lines demonstrate the confidence intervals of the several studies. Studies with greater populations typically have narrower confidence intervals. When the confidence interval line crosses the vertical line, it indicates that the study is not statistically significant.

The "blob" on each horizontal line represents the point estimate, the best guess of the true effect in the population. The area of the "blob" represents the size of the study, the number of individuals in the population studied.

The term "forest plot" seems to be inspired by the forest of horizontal lines in the plot. The term "blobbogram," on the other hand, focuses on the "blob" on each horizontal line.

The large diamond below the "forest" of horizontal lines represents the synthesis of the component studies. Its midpoint represents the point estimate, the best guess of the true effect in the combined population of all the studies.

The area of the diamond represents the number of individuals in the combined population of all the studies; hence, it is the largest enclosed area in the plot.

The width of the diamond represents the confidence interval for the overall effect estimate; hence, it is a short horizontal distance as the confidence interval narrows as the population considered increases.

Sometimes the large diamond representing the aggregate of the studies shows a statistical significance that the component studies do not. This demonstrates the **point of the meta-analysis, which is to accumulate a large enough population that a conclusion can be significantly drawn when the component studies are too small to support such an inference**.

The example forest plot below (Fig. 27.2) is from Wang's meta-analysis in the *Journal of Orthopedic Surgery and Research.* It concerns the effect of the use of fibrin sealant upon postoperative hemoglobin drop with total knee arthroplasty (Wang 2014), and exhibits some interesting features.

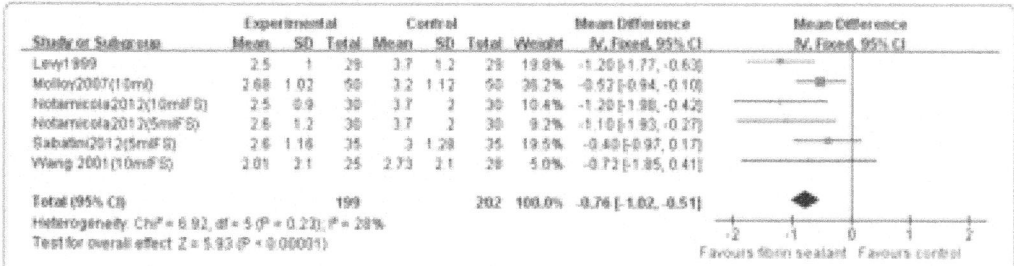

Figure 27.2 From Wang (2014). "Is fibrin sealant effective and safe in total knee arthroplasty? A meta-analysis of randomized trials." *Journal of Orthopaedic Surgery and Research*,9(1), 36.

The Molloy 2007 study has the largest population and the narrowest confidence interval. The Wang 2001 study has the smallest population and the widest confidence interval. The Wang 2001 study and the Sabatini 2012 studies exhibit confidence intervals that cross the vertical line of no effect, making those two studies not statistically significant.

The large diamond indicating total effect indicates that the most likely mean difference in hemoglobin drop is −0.76 points with a 95% confidence interval of -0.51 to -1.02 points. In other words, the patients treated with fibrin sealant most likely lost 0.76 grams of hemoglobin per deciliter (g/dl) less than the untreated patients with a 95% confidence interval of 0.51 g/dl to 1.02 g/dl.

Further information on interpreting forest plots is available in Gurusamy's *Interpretation of Forest Plots* and Sedgwick's *How to Read a Forest Plot in a Meta-analysis*.

Jadad Score

In 1996, **Jadad developed a simple system to rate the quality of a scientific or clinical study from 0 points (very poor) to 5 points (rigorous), based on three questions**. The questions must be answered "yes" or "no," and no fractional points are allowed.

The three questions and assigned points are as follows (Jadad 1996):
- Is the study described as randomized (including use of words such as "randomly," "random," and "randomization"? If "yes," assign one point. Is the randomization described and appropriate? If "yes," assign an additional point. If "no," delete all points for randomization.
- Is the study described as double-blinded? If "yes," assign one point. Is the double blinding described and appropriate? If "yes," assign an additional point. If "no," delete all points for blinding.
- Is there a description of reasons for withdrawals and dropouts? If "yes," assign one point. If there are no withdrawals or dropouts, it should be stated.

Additionally, Jadad cites a study by Colditz concluding that **non-randomized trials or randomized trials not using a double-blind design are more likely to show advantage of an innovation over standard treatment** (Colditz 1989). Jadad also points to a study of 250 trials from 33 meta-analyses showing that random controlled trials in which blinding was inadequate or unclear yielded significantly larger treatment effects than others in which blinding was adequate (Schulz 1995).

The Jadad Score represents a handy tool for use in critically evaluating the quality of medical studies.

Number Needed to Treat

A useful countermeasure to being deceived by misleading study conclusions is the calculation of the **number needed to treat (NNTT)**. Greenhalgh (Greenhalgh 1996, 2014) explains this concept by analyzing a study by Yusuf. This study compares the effects upon mortality of initial coronary artery bypass graft (CABG) surgery vs. initial medical therapy in patients with "stable coronary heart disease." The study defines "stable angina not severe enough to necessitate surgery on grounds of symptoms alone, or myocardial infarction" (Yusuf 1994).

The study randomized the patients into a group of 1325 who received medical therapy and 1324 who received CABG. At the end of 10 years, 404 of the medical group had died vs. 350 of the surgical group. The study concluded "initial CABG surgery is associated with lower mortality than one of medical management with delayed surgery if necessary."

In Greenhalgh's analysis, the medical group had an **absolute risk** of death in 10 years of 404/1325 or 30.5%. The CABG group had an **absolute risk** of death in 10 years of 350/1324 or 26.4%. Therefore, the **absolute risk reduction (ARR)** was 4.1% or 0.041. The **number needed to treat** in order to save one life is **1/ARR** = 1/0.041 = 24. Consequently, **24 patients with stable coronary artery disease must receive CABG in order to save one life over 10 years**.

Certainly, phrased in this way, the results do not seem nearly so impressive and one might imagine many patients declining the open-heart surgical option. One might also imagine many physicians answering differently if patients asked, "What would you do?"

Deaths from Any Cause

Deaths from any cause or all-cause mortality is an important statistic in evaluating a study. Firstly, **patients may suffer from comorbidities**. It does not benefit the patient to address one disease with a treatment that is painful, expensive, and debilitating when the patient harbors another disease expected to be fatal in the approximate same length of time. Secondly, the **treatment itself can have fatal adverse events** such that the patient becomes a victim of the treatment before becoming a victim of the disease.

A paradoxical conclusion that results when all-cause mortality is ignored is that **cigarette smoking reduces breast cancer mortality** by about one in one thousand women. This is actually true. However, the reason is that these women died from the results of cigarette smoking before they could become victims of breast cancer (Woloshin 2009, Gigerenzer 2015, p 213).

Let us proceed to examine some studies where all-cause mortality was significant.

Statin Study

Ray and colleagues acknowledged that statins reduce all-cause mortality in individuals *with a clinical history* of coronary heart disease; but, they determined to investigate if there was a similar mortality-reduction benefit in patients at high risk but still healthy (Ray 2010).

The Ray group conducted a meta-analysis of 11 randomized controlled trials (RCTs) involving 65,229 participants followed for 3.7 years. There were 1447 deaths occurring among 32,606 participants in the placebo groups and 1346 deaths among 32,623 participants in the statin-treated groups. The mean low-density lipoprotein cholesterol (LDL-C) levels were 134 mg/dL in the placebo groups compared with 94 mg/dL in the statins groups.

The Ray study was robust. It had 244,000 person-years of follow-up and seemed to have no substantial heterogeneity effect. There was no strong evidence of publication bias when assessed using a funnel plot. Additionally, as a measure against publication bias, the study incorporated unpublished tabular data from the incorporated studies.

This study found that the weighted mean rates for all-cause mortality were 11.4 per 1000 person-years in the placebo group vs. 10.7 per 1000 person-years in the statin-treated group. The difference was not statistically significant. The study also found no significant relationship between mean baseline levels of LDL-C and relative reduction in all-cause mortality in the studied population. Finally, the study failed to note any statistically significant correlation between statin-related difference in LDL-C levels and relative reduction in all-cause mortality

The Ray **study concluded that** over an average treatment period of 3.7 years, the use of **statin therapy did not result in reduction in all-cause mortality in those at high risk for coronary heart disease but without history of it.**

Fibrate Study

In 2007, Saha and colleagues published a systematic review and meta-analysis of randomized clinical trials evaluating the role of fibrates in the prevention of cardiovascular events (Saha 2007).

The Saha group's study involved 36,489 patients from 10 published randomized placebo-controlled trials. In this study, fibrates reduced plasma total cholesterol and triglyceride levels by about 8% and 30%, respectively, and raised high-density lipoprotein cholesterol levels by about 9% compared with placebo.

However, the odds of all-cause mortality tended to be higher ($P = .08$), and the odds of noncardiovascular mortality were significantly higher ($P = .004$) with the use of fibrates. While the higher fibrate mortality did not persist after exclusion of trials using clofibrate as the study drug, nevertheless fibrates did not significantly reduce the odds of cardiovascular mortality ($P = .68$), fatal myocardial infarction ($P = .76$), or stroke ($P = .56$). On the other hand, fibrates did significantly reduce the odds of nonfatal MI by about 22% ($P < .00001$).

Bevacizumab (Avastin™) Studies

Drug Description

Cancer drug **bevacizumab is a monoclonal antibody that binds to vascular endothelial growth factor (VEGF)** thus inhibiting the growth and maintenance of tumor blood vessels.

Bevacizumab's serious toxicities include hemorrhage, wound dehiscence and wound healing complications, gastrointestinal perforation, arterial thromboembolism, congestive heart failure, hypertension, proteinuria/nephrotic syndrome, infusion-related hypersensitivity reactions, and reversible posterior leukoencephalopathy syndrome (Gressett 2009).

Bevacizumab is currently indicated for metastatic colorectal cancer, some lung cancers, glioblastoma, metastatic renal cell carcinoma, recurrent carcinoma of the cervix, and recurrent ovarian cancer (Avastin 2017). However, the US Food and Drug Administration (US FDA) has withdrawn bevacizumab's indication for metastatic breast cancer (Hamburg 2011).

Drug Studies

In writing her report, FDA Commissioner Hamburg reviewed the submitted trials:
- The E2100 study (Miller 2007) was a randomized open-label trial that evaluated paclitaxel-plus-bevacizumab versus paclitaxel alone in metastatic breast cancer among 711 treated patients. While *progression-*

free survival in the paclitaxel-plus-bevacizumab group was 11.8 months, for paclitaxel alone it was 5.9 months. However, the *overall survival* (death from any cause) told a different story with 26.5 months in the paclitaxel-plus-bevacizumab group and 24.8 months in the paclitaxel-alone group. Further, no data were collected on adverse events that resulted in discontinuation of therapy.

- The AVF2119g study compared capecitabine-plus-bevacizumab against capecitabine-alone in 462 breast cancer patients. It found no statistically significant difference between the two groups in either progression-free survival or overall survival.
- The AVADO trial compared docetaxel-plus-bevacizumab against docetaxel-plus-placebo in 736 breast cancer (30.2com (patients. It found in the docetaxel-plus-bevacizumab group an increased progression-free survival (8.8 vs. 7.9 months) but a decreased overall survival (30.2 vs. 31.9 months).
- The RIBBON1 trial enrolled 1237 patients and showed favorable results for bevacizumab in progression-free survival but omitted data on overall survival in one of its two groups.
- The RIBBON2 study compared chemotherapy-plus-bevacizumab against chemotherapy-plus-placebo in 684 metastatic breast cancer patients (Brufsky 2011). It found advantage to the bevacizumab group in progression-free survival (7.2 vs. 5.1 months) but no statistically significant difference in overall survival. Importantly, an increased number of adverse events led to study discontinuation in the bevacizumab group (Hamburg 2011).

FDA Conclusion

In addition to the above data, the FDA also had access to quality-of-life assessments such as the questionnaire Functional Assessment of Cancer Therapy – Breast (FACT-B), not necessarily included in the journal publications. The FDA concluded that the above studies did not show improvement in quality of life measurements.

The FDA also cited adverse events, indicating that 1.7% of the 711 patients in the E2100 trial had deaths attributable to bevacizumab. The FDA indicated that of 2684 total patients in the studies E2100, AVADO, and RIBBON1, the chemotherapy-plus-bevacizumab groups had 1679 serious adverse events compared with 982 in the chemotherapy-alone groups. Frequency of adverse events was most notable for febrile neutropenia at 6.5% vs. 3.5%, hypertension at 9% vs. 1.2%, arterial thromboembolic events at 1.6% vs. 0.3%, hemorrhage at 1.5% vs. 0.4%, and abnormal tissue repair at 1.7% vs. 0.8%.

Finally, the FDA determined that the four succeeding studies did not substantiate the degree of progression-free survival suggested by the initial E2100 study.

The US FDA had, on February 22, 2008, given accelerated approval for bevacizumab with paclitaxel for metastatic breast cancer based on the first trial, the E2010, *under the condition that* additional studies be done to confirm benefit. However, the four succeeding studies did not verify benefit or show the drug to be safe and effective. Consequently, the FDA withdrew its conditional approval for metastatic breast cancer on November 18, 2011 (Hamburg 2011).

Afterthought

Some recurrent themes are associated with the five studies done in the case of bevacizumab.

- A number of the above studies were financed at least in part by the drug manufacturer.
- A number of the study authors had financial ties to the drug manufacturer.
- Study E2100 was an open label trial. It was thus subject to the type of *expectation bias* that double-blind studies were designed to counteract.
- It does not appear clear how dropouts were handled in the E2100 study. Dropouts are more frequently associated with treatment failure or side effects. If simply purged from the results, they often cause distortion of safety and effectiveness.
- Data omission in the published study is always a cause for concern.
- Surrogate outcomes such as progression-free survival may not reflect true outcomes.

Conclusion

In summary, countermeasures to misleading studies consist of skepticism toward industry-sponsored studies, searches for systematic reviews, consideration of forest plots or blobbograms, review of Jadad scores, calculation of number needed to treat and consideration of deaths from any cause. Finally, the absence of relevant information should be treated as disinformation. We expect, and our patients deserve, full disclosure.

References

Avastin (Bevacizumab): Side Effects, Interactions, Warning, Dosage & Uses. (n.d.). Retrieved October 19, 2017, from https://www.rxlist.com/avastin-drug.htm

Brufsky, A., Hurvitz, S., Perez, E., Swamy, R., Valero, V., O'Neill, V., & Rugo, H. (2011). RIBBON-2: a randomized, double-blind, placebo-controlled, phase III trial evaluating the efficacy and safety of bevacizumab in combination with chemotherapy for second-line treatment of human epidermal growth factor receptor 2-negative metastatic breast cancer. *Journal of Clinical Oncology,29*, 4286-4293. November 10, 2011

Cochrane. (n.d.). Retrieved August 31, 2017, from http://www.cochrane.org/

Colditz, G. A., Miller, J. N., & Mosteller, F. (1989). How study design affects outcomes in comparisons of therapy. I. Statistics in Medicine,8(4), 455-466. doi:10.1002/sim.4780080409

Gigerenzer, G. (2013). Better doctors, better patients, better decisions: envisioning health care 2020;. Cambridge, Mass.: MIT Press.

Gigerenzer, G. (2015). *Risk savvy: how to make good decisions*. London: Penguin Books.

Greenhalgh, T. (1996, 2014). How to read a paper: the basics of evidence based medicine. London: BMJ Books.

Gressett, S. M., & Shah, S. R. (2009). Intricacies of Bevacizumab-Induced Toxicities and Their Management. *Annals of Pharmacotherapy,43*(3), 490-501. doi:10.1345/aph.1I426

Gurusamy, K. (2017, September 14). Interpretation of Forest Plots - Part 1. Lecture presented at Interpretation of Forest Plots - Part 1, London, UK. Lecture - University College London

Hamburg, M., MD. (2011). *Proposal to Withdraw Approval for the Breast Cancer Indication for AVASTIN (Bevacizumab)*(USA, Food and Drug Administration, Office of the Commissioner). Washington, DC: US Government Printing Office. Docket No. FDA-2010-N-0621

Hedges, L. (1985). Statistical Methods for Meta-Analysis. Orlando, FL: Academic Press.

Jadad, A. R., Moore, R., Carroll, D., Jenkinson, C., Reynolds, D. M., Gavaghan, D. J., & Mcquay, H. J. (1996). Assessing the quality of reports of randomized clinical trials: Is blinding necessary? Controlled Clinical Trials,17(1), 1-12. doi:10.1016/0197-2456(95)00134-4

Kurkjian, C., & Kim, E. S. (2011). Risks and benefits with bevacizumab: evidence and clinical implications. *Therapeutic Advances in Drug Safety,3*(2), 59-69. doi:10.1177/2042098611430109

Miller, K., Wang, M., Gralow, J., Dickler, M., Cobleigh, M., Perez, E. A., . . . Davidson, N. E. (2007). Paclitaxel plus Bevacizumab versus Paclitaxel Alone for Metastatic Breast Cancer. *New England Journal of Medicine,357*(26), 2666-2676. doi:10.1056/nejmoa072113

Ranpura, V., Hapani, S., & Wu, S. (2011). Treatment-Related Mortality With Bevacizumab in Cancer Patients. Jama,305(5), 487. doi:10.1001/jama.2011.51

Ray, K., Seshasai, S., & Erqou, S. (2010). Statins and All-Cause Mortality in High-Risk Primary Prevention of Patients With Cardiovascular Risk Factors. *Archives of Internal Medicine,170*(22), 2041. doi:10.1001/archinternmed.2010.455

Saha, S. A., Kizhakepunnur, L. G., Bahekar, A., & Arora, R. R. (2007). The role of fibrates in the prevention of cardiovascular disease—a pooled meta-analysis of long-term randomized placebo-controlled clinical trials. *American Heart Journal,154*(5), 943-953. doi:10.1016/j.ahj.2007.07.011

Schulz, K. F. (1995). Empirical Evidence of Bias. JAMA,273(5), 408. doi:10.1001/jama.1995.03520290060030

Sedgwick, P. (2015, July 24). How to read a forest plot in a meta-analysis. Retrieved September 14, 2017, from http://www.bmj.com/content/351/bmj.h4028

Wang, H., Shan, L., Zeng, H., Sun, M., Hua, Y., & Cai, Z. (2014). Is fibrin sealant effective and safe in total knee arthroplasty? A meta-analysis of randomized trials. Journal of Orthopaedic Surgery and Research,9(1), 36. doi:10.1186/1749-799x-9-36

Woloshin, S., Schwartz, L. M., & Welch, H. G. (2009). Know your chances: understanding health statistics. Berkeley: University of California Press.

Yusuf, S., Zucker, D., Passamani, E., Peduzzi, P., Takaro, T., Fisher, L., . . . Chalmers, T. (1994). Effect of coronary artery bypass graft surgery on survival: overview of 10-year results from randomised trials by the Coronary Artery Bypass Graft Surgery Trialists Collaboration. The Lancet,344(8922), 563-570. doi:10.1016/s0140-6736(94)91963-1

Further Reading

Gigerenzer, G. (2013). Better doctors, better patients, better decisions: envisioning health care 2020;. Cambridge, Mass.: MIT Press.

Gigerenzer, G. (2015). *Risk savvy: how to make good decisions*. London: Penguin Books.

Goldacre, B. (2010). Bad science: quacks, hacks and big pharma -- flacks --. New York: Faber and Faber.

Goldacre, B. (2014). Bad pharma: how drug companies mislead doctors and harm patients. New York: Faber & Faber, Inc., an affiliate of Farrar, Straus and Giroux.

Greenhalgh, T. (2014). *How to Read a Paper: The Basics of Evidence-based Medicine*. Wiley-Blackwell.

Gurusamy, K. (2017, September 14). Interpretation of Forest Plots - Part 1. Lecture presented at Interpretation of Forest Plots - Part 1, London, UK. Lecture - University College London

Sedgwick, P. (2015, July 24). How to read a forest plot in a meta-analysis. Retrieved September 14, 2017, from http://www.bmj.com/content/351/bmj.h4028

Woloshin, S., Schwartz, L. M., & Welch, H. G. (2009). Know your chances: understanding health statistics. Berkeley: University of California Press.

Evaluating Medications

Chapter 28: Medications – Safety, Effectiveness, History, and Recommendations

Critical Thinking about Medications – Part One

Critical thinking about medications ... why is it necessary? Are there not laws rigidly regulating safety, effectiveness and labeling of medications? The surprising answer is that laws exist but that they are not nearly so long-established, so comprehensive, or so stringent as might be supposed. Consequently, every prescription written requires critical thinking about the safety and efficacy of the medications it specifies.

Let us begin with an examination of the three laws regulating the labeling, safety, and effectiveness of medications. The examination of these laws addresses their precise content as well as the events prompting their adoption.

First Step – Truth in Advertising

In the late 19th and early 20th century, regulation of food and drugs was virtually nonexistent. Coca-Cola contained significant amounts of cocaine (DEA [Drug Enforcement Administration] Museum.org 2017). The market was filled with products such as "Benjamin Bye's Soothing Balmy Oils to Cure Cancer" (Meadows 2016) and "Piso's Consumption Cure ... Cures Where All Else Fails" (Harper's Monthly, July 1881). Upton Sinclair exposed the situation in the meat packing industry in his book *The Jungle.* Samuel Hopkins Adams did the same for the patent medicine industry in a series of articles in *Collier's Weekly* (Adams 1907) and in the *Journal of the American Medical Association* (Adams 1914).

In response to the problem, Congress passed, and President Theodore Roosevelt signed, the **Wiley Act (Food and Drugs Act) of 1906**. The Wiley Act did not ensure the safety and effectiveness of medications. It **functioned mostly as a truth-in-labeling regulation**. The act required that if weights or amounts were indicated for the product, they had to be accurate. If contents were indicated, they had to be present. Finally, 11 specific adulterants, including alcohol, heroin, and cocaine, if present, had to be indicated, with amounts, on the label. Finally, the law could be invoked only if the product crossed state or national borders (USFDA - FDA's Origins and Functions – FDA History Part I 2009).

In 1917, under the Wiley Act, the US government in Rhode Island prosecuted Clark Stanley. The government based its case upon a report by the Secretary of Agriculture utilizing information from the Bureau of Chemistry. The federal prosecutors charged Stanley with misbranding because the department's analysis of **Clark Stanley Snake Oil Liniment** detected no snake oil. Crucially, Stanley was manufacturing the product in Rhode Island and selling it in Massachusetts. The prosecution succeeded. Mr. Stanley pleaded *nolo contendere* and paid a fine of $20 (Meadows 2006).

However, the limitations of the Wiley Act of 1906 were becoming clear as early as 1910. In that year, under the act, the US Government seized a medically ineffective product called Johnson's Mild Combination Treatment for Cancer. The government's case eventually reached the US Supreme Court, but the court ruled against the government. The court determined that the product's false claims of *effectiveness* were not within the scope of the Wiley Act (Meadows 2006).

To address the travesty of this 1910 US vs. Johnson decision, Congress passed the Sherley Amendment in 1912. This anemic amendment prohibited false therapeutic claims *if there was intent to defraud*. However, intent to defraud was difficult to prove, and false claims of efficacy, made in ignorance or faulty belief were still protected (Meadows 2006).

Such protection was demonstrated in the case of US vs. Leo Banks Barlett. Barlett was a shirt salesman from Pittsburgh who, in the late 1920s, began selling a **horsetail weed extract called Banbar as a cure for diabetes**. This occurred despite the fact that Sir Frederick Banting had discovered insulin in 1921 and that Lilly had brought it to market in 1923, the same year that Banting was awarded the Nobel Prize for its discovery. In the 1920s, insulin was already standard treatment.

From 1931 to 1933, the US government seized quantities of Banbar in several shipments from Pennsylvania to New York. It brought, under the Wiley Act, charges of mislabeling against Barlett, in the Federal Court of the Western District of Pennsylvania. The government introduced in evidence several deaths that resulted from public confidence in Banbar instead of insulin. However, not convinced that there was intent to defraud, the jury rendered a verdict of "not guilty" (FDA Notices of Judgment Collection, 1908-1966 2017).

Several more incidents illustrated the limitations of the Wiley Act. In 1933, over a **dozen women were blinded and one died from using permanent mascara named Lash Lure** (Committee to Update Science, Medicine, and Animals, National Research Council (n.d.), P. 21). This brought attention to the fact that cosmetics also needed regulation.

In 1932, **Eben Byers, steel mogul and Westinghouse Electric Board Member, died of radium poisoning**. Over a period of four and a half years, he had consumed 1400 bottles of the **patent medicine Radiothor, marketed mostly as a male potency enhancer** (Winslow 1990). Nevertheless, no case was possible; for, under the Wiley Act, the manufacturer was subject to prosecution only if the concoction did *not* contain the advertised radium and thorium. Clearly, new legislation was needed (Death Stirs Action on Radium 'Cures' 1932), but that legislation awaited one last high profile incident.

That incident finally came with the sulfanilamide elixir disaster. In 1935, the sulfanilamide antibiotic drug Prontosil was first used in the United States (Chandler 1950). It gained notoriety when it was used to treat the son of President Franklin Roosevelt in 1936 (Rubin 2007). However, Prontosil's limitation was poor solubility, which impeded its use in pediatric patients, who did not easily accept tablets or powders.

Then, in 1937, Harold Cole Watkins of **S. E. Massengill Company noted that sulfanilamide dissolved in diethylene glycol. Without testing for toxicity, the company prepared the formula as a raspberry flavored elixir** and sent 633 shipments around the country.

The first shipments were dispatched in early September. As soon as October 11, the American Medical Association (AMA) received reports of a new sulfanilamide preparation seeming to be involved in a number of deaths in Tulsa, Oklahoma. An AMA laboratory analyzed the preparation and isolated diethylene glycol, an already known poison. AMA began issuing radio and newspaper warnings.

On October 14, a New York physician alerted the Food and Drug Administration (FDA) to the danger. The FDA promptly identified the suspected deaths of eight children and one adult; it immediately dispatched inspectors to Massengill headquarters. The inspectors learned that Massengill had become aware of the situation and had sent telegrams to 1,000 salesmen, druggists, and doctors.

The telegrams, however, merely requested return of the product without mentioning the urgency and lethality of the situation. The FDA insisted on a second telegram. The company complied and the telegram read, "Imperative you take up all elixir sulfanilamide dispensed. Product may be dangerous to life. Return all stocks, our expense." Almost all of the shipped elixir was recovered, but not before **more than 100 people had died, many of them children**.

As a result of the deaths, the Massengill Company was fined $16,800. Remarkably, the penalty was for mislabeling. The label contained the word "elixir," which implied that the solvent ingredient was alcohol, when it was, in fact, diethylene glycol. Had the label read "solution" instead of "elixir," no charges could have been brought (Ballentine 1981, 2017).

Sixteen months after the first elixir shipments left Massengill headquarters, Harold Cole Watkins was found dead in his kitchen of a self-inflicted gunshot wound to the chest (Madera Tribune 1939).

Second Step – Medication Safety

The sulfanilamide elixir disaster, at last, catalyzed passage of the **1938 Food, Drug, and Cosmetic (FD&C) Act**. The new act **expanded regulation to cosmetics and medical devices and it required the manufacturer of a new drug to prove to the FDA the drug's safety before it could be sold** (US FDA - FDA's Origins and Functions - FDA History - Part II 2012).

However, the 1938 FD&C Act had two serious shortcomings. First, the FDA had only 60 days to prevent a new drug from going to market over safety concerns. Thereafter the drug could not be stopped. Second, drug manufacturers had only to prove safety, *not effectiveness* (USFDA, October 10, 2012). Harmless but worthless drugs were still permissible.

This changed with the **thalidomide event**. Thalidomide appeared on the German market in 1957 as the first non-barbiturate sedative and sleeping pill. It was considered safe, as no lethal dose for rats could be established. Thalidomide was soon being used in 46 countries. The US market had not yet been penetrated, but an application for marketing in the US had been submitted to the FDA (Fintel 2009).

Reviewing that application was physician and pharmacologist Frances Oldham Kelsey. In 1936, while a graduate student at the University of Chicago, she helped her mentor Eugene Geiling, who had been engaged by the FDA, in investigating the sulfanilamide elixir disaster.

Now, in September 1960, Dr. Kelsey had been working at the FDA for only one month when she was assigned the task of reviewing the Merrell Company's application for thalidomide. Kelsey examined the safety data submitted by the company and found it unsatisfactory, sometimes reading more like testimonials than scientific evidence. Consequently, she requested better data from the Merrell Company (US National Library of Medicine 2015, June 03; Kriplen 2017).

Kelsey was motivated by good science, not obstructionism. Although the manufacturer had repeatedly contacted her about progress on the application, Kelsey did not see the rush to approve a drug intended not for grave disease or intolerable suffering, but for sleeplessness. Additionally, she was suspicious that, although intended as a sleeping pill in humans, the drug did not seem to promote sleep in experimental animals (Mintz 1962). Finally, when she was at the University of Chicago during WWII working on a substitute for quinine for the government, she noted that quinine given to pregnant rabbits was metabolized well by the adults but killed the embryos. This made her curious about the effects of thalidomide upon the fetus (Kriplen 2017). She had good reason to request more data.

In early 1961, while awaiting the company's reply, Kelsey read in the *British Medical Journal* reports of possible thalidomide-related peripheral neuritis (Florence 1960). She noted that the Merrell Company had not mentioned this in the information the company had submitted. She requested still further details (Kriplen 2017).

Finally, while this was pending, there appeared in the December 16, 1961 issue of *The Lancet* a letter to the editor from Australian obstetrician W.G. McBride calling attention to a number of congenital deformities he had seen in the infants of mothers who had taken thalidomide during pregnancy. In the letter, McBride inquired of similar experiences from other physicians (McBride 1961).

At about the same time, West German pediatrician Widukind Lenz began making similar observations of congenital deformities. He informed the German manufacturer, Chemie Gruenenthal, by phone call of the problem on November 16, 1961 (Lenz 1992). Lenz also communicated this to *The Lancet* in a letter published January 6, 1962 (Lenz 1962).

Finally, on February 23, 1962, *Time* magazine, reported the Australian and European experiences in an article under "Medicine" entitled "Sleeping Pill Nightmare" (*Time*, 23 February 1962). Not surprisingly, in March 1962, Merrell withdrew its thalidomide application (Rice 2007).

The estimated **worldwide toll of the thalidomide disaster was 10,000 badly deformed infants** (Science Museum 2017) in addition to an unknown number of spontaneous abortions and stillbirths.

Third Step – Medication Effectiveness

The result of the thalidomide tragedy was a huge boost to passage of the **Kefauver-Harris Amendment** to the 1938 FD&C Act. Congress passed the Amendment and President John Kennedy **signed it into law on October 10, 1962** with Frances Kelsey in attendance.

The Kefauver-Harris Amendment substantially expanded the provisions of the 1938 FD&C Act. It required that
- Manufacturers prove not just the safety but also the effectiveness of drug products.
- manufacturers provide evidence based on well-controlled clinical studies not anecdotes.

- Studies obtain the informed consent of the subjects.
- FDA have 180 days to approve a new drug and that a new drug not be marketed without FDA approval.
- FDA conduct retrospective evaluations for effectiveness of drugs approved between 1938 and 1962.
- FDA take over control of drug advertising from the Federal Trade Commission (US Food and Drug Administration 2012).

The benefits of the Kefauver-Harris Amendment were soon evident. The **retrospective review for effectiveness of drugs that had been approved from 1938 until 1962 led to the withdrawal from market of 600 drugs** whose effectiveness could not be demonstrated (Green 2012).

Nevertheless, the give and take of politics made its mark upon the Amendment as finally passed. Kefauver initially wanted the Amendment to require not just effectiveness but comparative effectiveness. He wanted evidence that a new drug was not just effective but better than its predecessors (Green 2012).

Kefauver met with strong resistance in this. Disappointingly, even organized medicine resisted. The American Medical Association argued against the mandate of even ordinary effectiveness. It stated, "the only possible final determination as to the efficacy and ultimate use of a drug is the extensive clinical use of that drug by large numbers of the medical profession over a long period of time" (Green 2012, US Congress 1961). *The New England Journal of Medicine* argued only against the stronger comparative effectiveness provision, stating that proof of superiority was necessary only if superiority was actually claimed by the manufacturer (Green 2012, Ethical Drugs 1961).

Because of the resistance, comparative effectiveness had to be sacrificed in order to gain passage of the Amendment. Consequently, the adopted and presently existing measure of effectiveness of a medication is not comparison with other medications but comparison with a placebo. In brief, to be approved as effective, a medication does *not* need to show that it is better than other medications; it *only* needs to show that it is better than nothing! (Angell 2004, Kindle location 927 of 3627)

This disappointing situation is where we stand today.

Return to Critical Thinking about Medications

In conclusion, newly released drugs are not required to be as effective as their older, cheaper counterparts. In fact, they may be *less* effective. Additionally, the older medications have an information base capable of revealing possible long-term side effects, while newer medications lack this information base. No doubt, the writing of a prescription, especially for a new medication that has alternatives with broader background information, is a serious decision.

The question then arises, where do we turn for guidance in medication selection? The answer: **we must rely on our own critical awareness**.

This is a daunting challenge when direct-to-consumer ads on television and at every turn promote specific brands (availability bias), when well-dressed and well-groomed drug company representatives, "detail people," tirelessly hand out glossy "educational" materials to physicians (halo effect), or when many of one's peers are routinely prescribing the drug (conformity bias).

Faced with this challenge, it would be helpful to examine some of the **factors that comprise critical thinking in medication selection**.

- Are there head-to-head comparisons so that medications are compared to competing medications, not to placebos? Not surprisingly, pharmaceutical companies are not anxious to put their products at risk in such comparisons.
- If there are head-to-head comparisons, do they compare equivalent doses of the opposing drugs, or are they "loaded" by comparing maximum doses of one drug with minimum doses of another? (Angell 2004, Kindle location 963 of 3627)
- Are the comparisons double-blinded, so that neither the patients nor personnel administering the drugs know which drug the patient is receiving? This is necessary to minimize the influence of subtle subjective cues (expectation bias).
- Do the patients self-select for the two groups or are they selected in a truly random fashion? Is the random selection method specified?
- Are the comparisons crossover trials, so that each subject is given first one test preparation and then the other? In other words, does each subject try both test preparations?
- Do expert and disinterested parties make the comparisons, or do agents of the involved pharmaceutical companies make the comparisons?
- Are *all* of the results of the comparison published or are the results edited?
- Are there several independent comparison studies showing similar results? The FDA typically requires evidence that a drug worked better than placebo in two clinical trials, even if it did not in the other trials (Angell 1994; Angell 2004, Kindle location 1338 of 3627).
- If there are several comparison studies, are they truly independent or are they publications of different subsets of the same data creating the appearance of different independent studies?
- If all this information is not available, and it probably is not, then why not?

Very few drugs meet these standards, particularly, the standard of head-to-head comparison (Angell 2004, Kindle location 934 of 3627). Drug companies are reluctant to expose their heavily invested product to a do-or-die battle with another drug. Instead of specific primary efficacy, they prefer to compete on peripheral issues such as ease of swallowing or more convenient dosage schedule.

Nevertheless, evasion is not evidence, and neither are anecdotal narratives. Insufficient information, especially insufficient information on head-to-head comparisons, severely diminishes confidence in the choice of one drug over another.

Finally, if one drug is proven truly superior to another, does the degree in superiority justify the price difference? Consideration must be given to the fact that the expenditure difference between two drugs consumes resources available for prevention, diagnosis, treatment, and other medications.

Conclusion

Critical thinking is a central obligation in all of medical decision-making. It should never be abandoned in the mistaken belief that omniscient government authorities or selfless pharmaceutical manufacturers have already addressed these issues.

References

Adams, S. H. (1907). The Great American Fraud (4th ed.). Chicago`, Illinois: Press of American Medical Association.
ARTICLES ON THE NOSTRUM EVIL AND QUACKS REPRINTED FROM COLLIER'S WEEKLY

Adams, S. H. (1914). Do Patent Medicines Control the Press? An Example. Journal of the American Medical Association,LXIII(23), 2062. doi:10.1001/jama.1914.02570230072029

Angell, M. (2004). The truth about the drug companies: how they deceive us and what to do about it. New York City, NY: Random House. Kindle location 963 of 3627

Angell, M., & Kassirer, J. P. (1994). Clinical Research -- What Should the Public Believe? New England Journal of Medicine,331(3), 189-190. doi:10.1056/nejm199407213310309

Ballentine, C. (1981, June). Sulfanilamide Disaster. Retrieved June 08, 2017, from https://www.fda.gov/AboutFDA/WhatWeDo/History/ProductRegulation/Sulfanilam ideDisaster/default.htm

FDA Consumer magazine - June 1981 Issue

Cannabis, Coca, & Poppy: Nature's Addictive Plants. (n.d.). Retrieved June 06, 2017, from https://www.deamuseum.org/ccp/coca/history.html

Chandler, C. A. (1950). Famous Men of Medicine . New York, NY: Dodd, Mead & Co.

Chemist of Death Elixir Is Suicide. (1939, January 18). Madera Tribune, Number 64. Body Found in Home with Bullet Wound.

Committee to Update Science, Medicine, and Animals, National Research Council. (n.d.). Science, Medicine, and Animals. The National Academies Press. doi:10.17226/10733

DEATH STIRS ACTION ON RADIUM 'CURES' (1932, April 02). New York Times.

Dove, F. (2011, November 03). What's happened to Thalidomide babies? Retrieved June 15, 2017, from http://www.bbc.co.uk/news/magazine-15536544

Ethical Drugs — Reflections on the Inquiry. (1961). New England Journal of Medicine,265(20), 1015-1016. doi:10.1056/nejm196111162652013

FDA Notices of Judgment Collection, 1908-1966. (n.d.). Retrieved June 07, 2017, from https://ceb.nlm.nih.gov/fdanj/handle/123456789/57283

FDA's Origin & Functions - FDA History - Part I. (2009, June 18). Retrieved June 09, 2017, from https://www.fda.gov/AboutFDA/WhatWeDo/History/Origin/ucm054819.htm

Fintel, B., Samaras, A., & Carias, E. (2009, July 28). Helix Magazine: The Thalodimide Tragedy: Lessons for Drug Safety and Regulation. Retrieved June 09, 2017, from https://helix.northwestern.edu/article/thalidomide-tragedy-lessons-drug-safety-and-regulation

Florence, A. L. (31 December 1960). Is Thalidomide to Blame? British Medical Journal,2(5217), 1954-1954. doi:10.1136/bmj.2.5217.1954

Greene, J. A., & Podolsky, S. H. (18 october 2012). Reform, Regulation, and Pharmaceuticals — The Kefauver–Harris Amendments at 50. New England Journal of Medicine,367(16), 1481-1483. doi:10.1056/nejmp1210007

Kriplen, N. (2017, February 06). The Heroine of the FDA. Discover Magazine.

Lenz, W. (1962). Thalidomide and Congenital Abnormalities. The Lancet,199-199. doi:10.1007/978-94-011-6621-8_28
Letter to the Editor, 6 January 1962

Lenz, W. (1992). THE HISTORY OF THALIDOMIDE by Dr. Widukind Lenz. Lecture presented at UNITH Congress 1992.

Mcbride, W. (1961). Thalidomide And Congenital Abnormalities. The Lancet,278(7216), 1358. doi:10.1016/s0140-6736(61)90927-8

Meadows, M. (2006, February). Centennial Edition of FDA Consumer - Promoting Safe and Effective Drugs for 100 Years. Retrieved June 06, 2017, from https://www.fda.gov/AboutFDA/WhatWeDo/History/CentennialofFDA/Centennial EditionofFDAConsumer/ucm093787.htm

Mintz, M. (1962, July 15). 'Heroine" of FDA Keeps Bad Drug off Market. The Washington Post.

Neeley, K. L. (n.d.). Frances Kathleen Oldham Kelsey. Retrieved June 11, 2017, from http://www.chemistryexplained.com/Hy-Kr/Kelsey-Frances-Kathleen-Oldham.html
Piso's Consumption Cure ,,, Cures Where Al Else Fails. (1881, July). Harper's Monthly.
Advertisement

Rice, E. L. (2007). Dr. Frances Kelsey: Turning the Thalidomide Tragedy into Food and Drug Administration Reform(Unpublished doctoral dissertation).

Rubin, R. P. (2007). A Brief History of Great Discoveries in Pharmacology: In Celebration of the Centennial Anniversary of the Founding of the American Society of Pharmacology and Experimental Therapeutics. Pharmacological Reviews,59(4), 289-359. doi:10.1124/pr.107.70102

Science Museum. Brought to Life: Exploring the History of Medicine. (n.d.). Retrieved June 15, 2017, from www.sciencemuseum.org.uk/broughttolife/themes/controversies/thalidomide
Funded by: The Wellcome Trust

Sleeping Pill Nightmare. (1962, February 23). Time Magazine, 86-87.

Tabler, D. (2016, October 06). My Chemists and I Deeply Regret the Fatal Results. Retrieved June 08, 2017, from http://www.appalachianhistory.net/
Appalachian History Stories, quotes and anecdotes.

U.S.Cong. (1961). Drug Industry Antitrust Act[Cong. Bill from 87th Cong., 1st sess.

U.S. Food and Drug Administration. (2009, June 18). FDA's Origin & Functions - FDA History - Part I. Retrieved June 09, 2017, from https://www.fda.gov/AboutFDA/WhatWeDo/History/Origin/ucm054819.htm

U.S. Food and Drug Administration. (2012, September 24). FDA's Origin & Functions - FDA History - Part II The 1938 Food, Drug, and Cosmetic Act. Retrieved June 9, 2017, from www.fda.gov/AboutFDA/WhatWeDo/History/Origin/ucm054819.htm

U.S. Food and Drug Administration. (2012, October 10). Consumer Updates - Kefauver-Harris Amendments Revolutionized Drug Development. Retrieved June 09, 2017, from https://www.fda.gov/ForConsumers/ConsumerUpdates/ucm322856.htm

US National Library of Medicine. (2015, June 03). Changing the Face of Medicine | Frances Kathleen Oldham Kelsey. Retrieved June 10, 2017, from https://cfmedicine.nlm.nih.gov/physicians/biography_182.html

Winslow, R. (1990, August 1). The Radium Water Worked Fine until His Jaw Came Off. The Wall Street Journal.

Further Reading

Angell, M. (2004). The truth about the drug companies: how they deceive us and what to do about it. New York City, NY: Random House.

Chapter 29: Medications: Off-Label Advertising

Critical Thinking about Medications – Part Two

The last chapter presented the necessity of thinking critically about medications given the circumscribed power of laws regarding labeling, safety, and effectiveness of medications. This chapter presents the **necessity of thinking critically about medications given the legal status of off-label drug advertising** and the sometimes-unreliable manufacturers' claims of conditions treated by their medications.

A helpful start would be an examination of the law regarding off-label use.

Kefauver-Harris Amendment 1962

Recall from the previous chapter that the 1962 Kefauver-Harris Amendment to the 1938 FD&C Act was passed by Congress and signed into law by President John Kennedy. The Amendment required that before being allowed to market a new drug, the manufacturer had to provide to the Food and Drug Administration (FDA) "substantial evidence of effectiveness *for the product's intended use* (italics mine)" (Meadows 2006).

In other words, the **FDA requires specification of the disease or condition upon which the medication has been tested and for which it is therefore approved**. These approved conditions are displayed in the medication information as "labeled uses." The FDA approval includes both the medication *and* the label (O'Reilly 2003). The manufacturer or distributor may promote the drug only for the conditions listed on the label.

However, **once the FDA has approved a medication as safe and effective for a given condition, a physician is free to prescribe it for another condition if so determined in his or her critical medical judgment**. This other condition could be one for which the patient tolerates no other treatment or for which no other treatment is available. Such a medication use is called "off-label."

In permitting off-label uses of a drug but prohibiting off-label advertising of the same drug, the Food and Drug Administration (FDA) has sought to strike a balance between recognizing the ability of physicians to prescribe according to their best clinical judgment and preventing drug manufacturers from inappropriately influencing prescribing practices. The FDA has long maintained the position that although physicians may freely prescribe drugs for off-label uses, drug manufacturers may not promote such uses (Mello 2009).

Fen-Phen Off-Label Tragedy

Fen-Phen was not a single preparation, but rather the practice of **off-label prescribing phentermine in the morning and fenfluramine in the evening for weight reduction**. The FDA had independently approved fenfluramine in 1973 and phentermine in 1959, each for *short-term* appetite suppression. In 1979, fenfluramine was patented as Pondimin™ by American Home Products, which later became Wyeth. Meanwhile, phentermine had been out of patent.

In the 1980s, at the University of Rochester, Dr. Michael Weintraub considered the possibility that since fenfluramine and phentermine had different mechanisms of action they might act *synergistically* rather than simply *additively*. They might therefore suppress appetite substantially better than expected. He also considered the possibility that, since obesity is a chronic disease, it might need to be treated long-term with this combination (Kolata 1993) (Cohen 2003).

Weintraub conducted a double-blind study of 121 people over 34 weeks. It compared 60 mg of extended-release fenfluramine plus 15 mg phentermine resin against placebo. Both groups received behavior modification, calorie restriction, and exercise. The **fen-phen group lost an average 15.9% +/- 0.9% body weight versus 4.9% +/- 0.9% for the placebo group (Weintraub** [weeks 0 to 34] 1992).

Weintraub also did a double-blind study of 52 participants over almost four years using the same experimental and control conditions. He found that at week 190, although both groups had regained some weight, both were still below their initial weight. The fenfluramine-phentermine group regained 5.3% +/- 0.5% of initial weight while the control group regained 8.5% +/- 1.0% (Weintraub [weeks 156 to 190] 1992).

Weintraub published these studies in 1992 in *Clinical Pharmacology and Therapeutics*. Reprints of the articles found quick dissemination (Mundy 2001), and **physicians began the off-label prescription of fenfluramine with phentermine** for their patients (Cohen 2003).

Meantime, in 1995, Wyeth introduced dexfenfluramine, the dextrorotary component of fenfluramine, which it marketed as Redux™. The technical rationale for dexfenfluramine was that it might not be so sedating as fenfluramine. The economic rationale was that the patent for fenfluramine was expiring.

Physicians now began the off-label prescription of dexfenfluramine and phentermine. In 1996, there were over 18 million prescriptions for the combination of dexfluramine and phentermine (Cohen 2003) (Connolly 1997).

However, in 1996, at Mayo Clinic, Dr. Heidi Connolly and her associates began noticing cases in which the pathological findings on surgically removed, diseased cardiac valves seemed identical to findings of valvular fibrosis in carcinoid syndrome, methylsergide use, and ergotamine use. However, the afflicted patients had no history of carcinoid, methylsergide, or ergotamine. They did, however, have a history of fen-phen.

Dr. Connolly's suspicions intensified in January 1997 with an inquiry from cardiologist Dr. Jack Crary in Fargo, ND. Dr. Crary, alerted by echocardiographer Pam Ruff, had noted unusual echocardiographic findings in 12 patients, all having reported a history of fen-phen treatment (Connolly 1997) (Mundy 2001).

In August 1997, Dr. Connolly and the **Mayo group published a study in *The New England Journal of Medicine* reporting 24 cases of echocardiographic evidence of unusual cardiac valvular disease**, identical to that seen in carcinoid and ergotamine exposure. The 24 patients, all women, had been on fen-phen for anywhere from one to 28 months. All were thought to be free of cardiovascular disease at the onset of weight-reduction treatment.

Twenty of the patients had the echocardiography because of cardiovascular symptoms and four had it because of murmur. Eight of the patients had Doppler or catheter evidence of pulmonary hypertension that had not been previously documented. Five of the 24 required cardiac surgery to address their damaged heart valves.

The age of the group (mean +/- SD) was 44 +/- 8 years. The rarity of left sided regurgitant valvular heart disease in a population less than 50 years of age, along with the unusual echocardiographic morphology of the lesions, made coincidence highly unlikely (Connolly 1997).

Because of the findings at the Mayo Clinic, and **another 75 cases of heart valve disease reported to the FDA in 1997**, both Pondimin™ (fenfluramine) and Redux™ (dexfenfluramine) were withdrawn from the market on Sept. 15, 1997 (Cohen 2003).

Cardiac valvular fibrosis and primary pulmonary hypertension are potentially fatal conditions sometimes amenable to treatment with cardiac valve replacement and lung transplantation, respectively. They are costly in both human suffering and economic terms. By 2005, according to the *New York Times*, **Wyeth had set aside $21.1 billion to cover litigation reserves for the fen-phen cases** involving Pondimin™ and Redux™ (Saul 2005).

Fen-Phen – What Went Wrong

To be fair, the thinking of the physicians involved in the fen-phen tragedy may have been that the safety of fenfluramine and phentermine was not in doubt. After all, the drugs had already been on the market. Nevertheless, this supposition was wrong.

The error was that just as drugs are *effective* for specific conditions, in specific types of patients, at specific doses, and for specific durations, so also they are *safe* for specific conditions, in specific types of patients, at specific doses, and for specific durations. **The fact that a drug has been approved for market under specific conditions does not mean that it is universally safe**.

The critical test of safety as well as effectiveness is whether the drug or treatment survives the challenge of stringent studies that are conceived critically, executed without bias and on large representative population samples, analyzed appropriately, reported accurately, and replicated by independent researchers. This did not happen in Weintraub's fen-phen study.

Instead, the assumption that the drugs were universally safe and worthy of use on resistant obesity was based on the biases of action, availability, confirmation, and novelty.

The planning bias also played a major part in the error, indeed, in two ways.

First, the idea of safe use was so intensely ingrained that there were **not even animal studies done to substantiate the safety of the fen-phen plan** (Wellman 1999).

Second, the idea was captivating that the different mechanisms of action of fenfluramine and phentermine would allow them to combine for weight loss synergistically rather than simply additively. It was sufficiently captivating to **exclude from consideration the possibility that side effects could also combine synergistically rather than simply additively**. The role of synergism in the damaging side effects of pulmonary vasoconstriction and valvular disease was later elucidated by Wellman and Maher (Wellman 1999).

Government Actions against Promotion of Drugs for Off-Label Uses

Following the fen-phen debacle, the government took aggressive action against manufacturers that promoted their drugs for off-label uses. Some examples are noteworthy.

Zyprexa

Zyprexa™ is the brand name for olanzapine, a drug developed by Elli Lilly & Co. and FDA-cleared to market for the treatment of schizophrenia and bipolar disorder. Nevertheless, between September 1999 and March 2001 Lilly marketed the drug for the treatment of a different condition, dementia, including Alzheimer's-related dementia (Eli Lilly Settles Zyprexa 2009).

In January 2009, Lilly & Co. said that it pleaded guilty and would pay $1.43 billion to settle civil suits and end the criminal investigation. Of the $1.43 billion, $438 million was allocated to the federal government in civil suits, $362 million was allocated to states in civil suits, and $615 million was allocated to resolve the criminal probe (NBC News January 2009).

Laurie Majid, federal prosecutor in the case, asserted that the public has an absolute right to know that their doctor's judgment "has not been clouded by misinformation from a company trying to build its bottom line" (US Department of Justice January 2009). She emphasized that off-label marketing circumvents "the very process put in place to protect the public" (NBC News 2009).

Actiq

Actiq™, produced by the pharmaceutical company Caphalon, is a formulation of fentanyl, a narcotic analgesic, often considered 100 times more potent than morphine. The **FDA had approved Actiq only for the treatment of opioid-tolerant cancer patients**.

Nevertheless, according to the US Department of Justice's report, Cephalon, between 2001 and 2006, promoted the drug for use in such maladies as migraines, sickle-cell pain crises, injuries, and in anticipation of changing wound dressings or radiation therapy. **Cephalon also promoted Actiq for use with patients who were not opioid tolerant**.

The US Attorney's Office in Philadelphia, the Justice Department's Civil Division, and the FDA's Office of Criminal Investigation brought charges of marketing for unapproved uses. As a result, in 2008, Cephalon agreed to enter a criminal plea and pay $425 million to resolve claims that it had illegally marketed Actiq and two other drugs.

Of the $425 million penalty, $40 million was applied to a criminal fine. Another $375 million, plus interest, went toward resolving False Claims Act allegations arising from claims to Medicaid, Medicare, and other federal programs. Finally, $116 million went toward resolving False Claims Act allegations involving state Medicaid programs in 13 states and the District of Columbia (Criminal Investigations FDA 2008).

Bextra

Bextra™ (valdecoxib) was a nonsteroidal anti-inflammatory drug (NSAID) made by Pfizer and approved by the FDA in 2001 specifically for the treatment of osteoarthritis, rheumatoid arthritis, and dysmenorrhea. Nevertheless, **Pfizer promoted the sale of Bextra for several uses and dosages that the FDA specifically declined to approve due to safety concerns. Bextra was pulled from the market in 2005**.

According to the plea arrangement with the US Department of Justice, Pfizer agreed to pay $1.3 billion in criminal fines and $1 billion to resolve civil allegations under the False Claims Act for illegally promoting Bextra and three other drugs (Justice Department 2009).

Promoting Off-Label Drug Promotion

Despite the fen-phen tragedy, the push for expansion of off-label drug and device marketing continues. **Distribution of reprints of medical journal articles describing unapproved uses of drugs and devices has already been permitted by the FDA guidelines of 2009**. Currently on the horizon is marketing of off-label uses to the public by direct-to-consumer (DTC) advertising.

Proponents of off-label drug and device promotion offer several reasons why they think such promotion would be beneficial. They argue
* It would allow more data to be readily available to prescribers.
* It is nearly impossible for a physician to read all the medical journals and compendia.
* It would reduce the delay and cost associated with the FDA's drug approval process.
* It would allow drug manufacturers to keep research and development costs down, while still gaining the revenue from off-label sales.
* It would benefit Americans suffering from orphan diseases.
* It would expedite accessibility to new treatments (O'Reilly and Dalal 2003).

It seems, however, that all of these arguments have one thing is common; they all assume that the information conveyed by off-label promotion would always be correct. Nevertheless, if it is not, then the greater availability of untested drugs and treatments, at best, accelerates a waste of time, money, and resources, and, at worst, speeds the path to patient harm or death.

Further, drug manufacturers have a direct financial stake in the commercial success of their products. Consequently, information being disseminated by the manufacturers has a greater chance of being biased and a greater chance of being misleading (O'Reilly and Dalal 2003).

Danger of Off-Label Drug Promotion

Off-label drug promotion is destructive of the very idea of drug regulation.

First, off-label promotion conduces to bypassing the safety and effectiveness safeguards so painstakingly established by the 1938 Food, Drug, and Cosmetic Act and its successors. **Allowing the distribution of off-label reprints permits manufacturers to go directly to physicians with new uses when they might otherwise have conducted clinical trials** to seek approval for them (Ventola 2009).

Second, **off-label promotion is a disincentive for manufacturers to perform clinical trials**. Manufacturers conducting such clinical studies may learn that their intended off-label use is ineffective or harmful, and thus may be prohibited from promotion or sale (O'Reilly and Dalal 2003). Indeed, **it may be profitable for manufacturers not to know of adverse effects**.

Third, **off-label promotion of drugs may encourage manufacturers to seek FDA approval only for the narrowest and easiest-to-prove uses**, knowing that they can then advertise the product for a wide variety of applications (Ventola 2009).

Legal Future of Off-Label Advertising

Despite the past aggressive actions of the US Justice Department against off-label promotion of medications, the fate of off-label promotion by pharmaceutical manufacturers is anything but sealed.

FDA 2009 Guidelines

FDA guidelines issued January 2009 seemed to backpedal. They explicitly allowed drug and device manufacturers to distribute reprints of peer-reviewed medical journal articles that described unapproved uses of drugs and devices so long as they were not "false or misleading" and were published in a reputable journal (Mello 2009) (Guidance for Industry – Federal Register 2009) (Guidance for Industry – FDA n.d.).

Nevertheless, reliance on a journal's reputation and supposed ability to detect fraud is a poor warrant for confidence in the conclusions of a study. Flawed and fraudulent studies often find their way into reputable journals. If these are detected, reputable journals retract them. In fact, 2,047 articles were listed as retracted by PubMed as of May 3, 2012 (Fang 2012). This testifies to the frequency of the problem. Journal editors, publishers, and readers have often been fooled despite their apparent expertise and good intentions.

Additionally, there were other significant points on which the 2009 FDA guidelines seemed lax compared to the preceding 1997 FDA Modernization Act. Notably,

- There was no mention that the drug or device must have received prior FDA approval for *some* use, however unrelated.
- There was no mention that the manufacturer must have submitted a supplemental application for the proposed new use. This is important because a supplemental application needs to supply as much evidence of safety and effectiveness for the new use as the original application did for the original use.
- There was no mention that the manufacturer must have submitted the promotional materials to the FDA prior to dissemination (Mello 2009).

The relaxed 2009 FDA guidelines may have resulted from the following adverse Supreme Court ruling.

Thompson v. Western State Medical Center

A Supreme Court decision in 2002 affirmed that drug advertising is entitled to First Amendment protection as commercial speech (Mello 2009) (Thompson v. Western States Medical Center 2002).

Tommy Thompson is listed as one of the litigants in the case because he was, at the time, US Secretary of Health and Human Services. The other litigant, Western States Medical Center, was a group of licensed pharmacies that specialized in compounding drugs.

Compounding pharmacies prepare pharmaceuticals in small batches from basic ingredients. They differ from dispensing pharmacies, which retail pharmaceuticals that are prepared at a factory in large batches. Compounding pharmacies often create individual preparations for patients who require dosages or dosage forms not available "off the shelf." Compounding pharmacies may serve a patient intolerant to certain inactive ingredients such as colors common in "off the shelf" medications. They do this by compounding a custom preparation without the offending ingredient. Because compounding pharmacies may prepare unique products for select individuals, their preparations can be regarded as off-label.

The Western States compounding pharmacists sought to enjoin enforcement of the advertising and solicitation subsections of the stringent 1997 Act. They argued that those provisions violated the First Amendment's free speech guarantee. The District Court agreed and granted their motion for summary judgment.

On appeal, the Ninth Circuit Court agreed with the District Court that the 1997 Act's restrictions regarding advertisement and promotion were unconstitutional. The case made its way to the United States Supreme Court. On April 29, 2002, Justice Sandra Day O'Connor handed down the Court's decision. The US Supreme Court affirmed the Appeals Court's judgment that the provisions regarding off-label advertisement and promotion amounted to unconstitutional restrictions on commercial speech (Thompson v. Western States Medical Center 2002).

These **commercial free speech judicial decisions are especially concerning as they could strengthen the position of off-label drug advertising *direct to consumers via television and magazine ads***.

Finally, the aforementioned free speech judicial decisions could switch the issue of off-label drug promotion from the criminal arena to the civil arena.

Criminal vs. Civil

The difference between criminal and civil liability became clear to many of us during the two trials of O. J. Simpson. In 1995, in a criminal trial, O. J. Simpson was acquitted of the 1994 murders of Nicole Brown Simpson and Ronald Goldman. However, in 1997, in a civil trial, Simpson was found responsible for both deaths and was ordered to pay $33.5 million in compensatory and punitive damages to the Brown and Goldman families.

Civil as well as criminal penalties emerged in the aforementioned cases of Zyprexa, Actiq, and Bextra. In these cases, the dollar amount of the civil penalties approached or exceeded that of the criminal penalties.

While commercial free speech protections may insulate off-label marketing of drugs from criminal penalties, they do not provide protection from the civil consequences of resulting injuries. In fact, if decreased criminal penalties lead to increased off-label promotion, and increased off-label promotion leads to increased prescription with concomitant injurious consequences, then increased judicial civil actions can be expected to result.

Importantly, increased off-label promotion and increased judicial civil actions markedly change the situation for physicians.

Increased Civil Liability for Physicians

Increased civil liability for physicians could emerge from increased off-label drug promotion for two reasons.

First, the fact remains that some physicians will uncritically accept the poorly tested claims of off-label marketing and initiate therapy that results in injury and civil claims.

Second, when a patient is injured by the off-label use of a product, he or she will typically file a product liability claim against the manufacturer and a malpractice claim against the doctor. These dual claims often lead to a battle of the defendants at trial, where each side blames the other for the resulting injury. The manufacturer claims the doctor's use was not foreseeable by the manufacturer, while the doctor claims that such use was one commonly engaged in by the profession and sanctioned by the manufacturer (O'Reilly and Dalal 2003).

In short, the relaxation of limitations against off-label drug promotion could well result in physicians finding themselves increasingly involved in liability suits, with courtroom accusations coming from both patients and drug manufacturers.

Increased Physician Responsibility as Seen by the Court

In 1993, the Washington Legal Foundation (WLF) filed a lawsuit in the District Court for the District of Columbia against Michael Friedman, MD, as the Acting Commissioner of the FDA and against Donna Shalala, as the Secretary of Health and Human Services.

The suit claimed that the FDA's off-label policies infringed on the First Amendment rights of WLF members. In 1997, after the discovery phase, Judge Royce C. Lamberth, ruled against the FDA and granted WLF's motion for summary judgment and permanent injunction against the FDA (Washington Legal Foundation v. Friedman 1998).

Following this ruling, it became common for pharmaceutical companies to send out journal reprints describing the off-label use of drugs, accompanied by the suggested disclosure that the usage had not received FDA approval. The FDA did not attempt to stop the distribution (Mello 2009).

The central issue of this case was that speech is afforded more constitutional protection than is conduct, and that FDA regulation of off-label promotion was a regulation of speech, not conduct. Specifically, Judge Lamberth ruled that the "court is hard pressed to believe that the agency [FDA] is seriously contending that 'promotion' of an activity is conduct and not speech."

Nevertheless, Judge Lamberth qualified his ruling, stating that the court's decision in no way hindered the FDA from restricting claims that are *actually* false and misleading (Washington Legal Foundation v. Friedman 1998) (O'Reilly and Dalal 2003). Unfortunately, off-label promotion such as distribution of reprints easily evades this requirement by third party attribution of claims.

The outcome of this is that the critical evaluation of off-label promotion falls to the physician. The **court rejected the FDA's argument that "most physicians, well-educated and experienced though they may be, do not have the resources, experience, or education to critically evaluate evidence concerning off-label uses."** Instead, the court held that the government could not regulate off-label "speech" out of fear of misuse by physicians (Washington Legal Foundation v. Friedman 1998).

The **court further stated, "A physician's livelihood depends upon the ability to make accurate, life-and-death decisions based upon the scientific evidence before them. They are certainly capable of critically evaluating journal articles or textbook reprints** that are mailed to them, or the findings presented at CME [Continuing Medical Education] seminars."

Finally, the court stated that it was unclear "why the ability of a doctor to critically evaluate scientific findings depends upon how the article got into the physician's hands, or whether a manufacturer suggests speakers or content for a CME [Continuing Medical Education] seminar" (Washington Legal Foundation v. Friedman 1998).

Conclusion

In summary, physicians are being held to a high level of responsibility in critically evaluating information presented to them. Society expects physicians to act on evidence, not hearsay. The public trust is poorly served when physicians allow themselves to be gulled and guiled by special interests and commercial influences. The physician's role consists in critically evaluating evidence and acting appropriately on that which is truly legitimate. Physicians cannot abandon this professional responsibility and instead blindly implement the latest therapy suggested to them by entities with priorities other than public health. The public entrusts their lives and well being to the physician's critical medical judgment. The physician must not fail this trust.

References

Cohen, K. (Writer). (2003, November 13). Fen-Phen Nation[Radio broadcast]. In Frontline - Dangerous Prescription. Erie, Pennsylvania: PBS - WQLN.

Commissioner, O. O. (2009, January). Search for FDA Guidance Documents - Good Reprint Practices for the Distribution of Medical Journal Articles and Medical or Scientific Reference Publications on Unapproved New Uses of

Approved Drugs and Approved or Cleared Medical Devices. Retrieved January 26, 2018, from
https://www.fda.gov/RegulatoryInformation/Guidances/ucm125126.htm

Connolly, H. M., Crary, J. L., Mcgoon, M. D., Hensrud, D. D., Edwards, B. S., Edwards, W. D., & Schaff, H. V. (1997). Valvular Heart Disease Associated with Fenfluramine–Phentermine. New England Journal of Medicine,337(9), 581-588. doi:10.1056/nejm199708283370901

Criminal Investigations - September 29, 2008: Pharmaceutical Company Cephalon to Pay $425 Million for Off-label Drug Marketing. Retrieved January 16, 2018, from https://www.fda.gov/ICECI/CriminalInvestigations/ucm260715.htm

Fang, F. C., Steen, R. G., & Casadevall, A. (2012). Misconduct accounts for the majority of retracted scientific publications. Proceedings of the National Academy of Sciences,109(42), 17028-17033. doi:10.1073/pnas.1212247109

GUIDANCE FOR INDUSTRY - Food and Drug Administration. (n.d.). Retrieved January 18, 2018, from
https://www.bing.com/cr?IG=852B48FCF89A42DA9E89D3BA5B05390D&CID=18410E93184F6BBD244E05E819E06AB6&rd=1&h=H6AYL2O9ed0okh3a8FO7R2pUKAxFLTPUf_zw3GsN_JI&v=1&r=https%3a%2f%2fwww.fda.gov%2fohrms%2fdockets%2f98fr%2ffda-2008-d-0053-gdl.pdf&p=DevEx,5067.1

Guidance for Industry on Good Reprint Practices for the Distribution of Medical Journal Articles and Medical or Scientific Reference Publications on Unapproved New Uses of Approved Drugs and Approved or Cleared Medical Devices; Availability. (2009, January 13). Retrieved January 18, 2018, from https://www.federalregister.gov/documents/2009/01/13/E9-452/guidance-for-industry-on-good-reprint-practices-for-the-distribution-of-medical-journal-articles-and

Justice Department Announces Largest Health Care Fraud Settlement in Its History. (2009, September 02). Retrieved January 17, 2018, from https://www.justice.gov/opa/pr/justice-department-announces-largest-health-care-fraud-settlement-its-history

Kolata, G. (1997, September 23). How FenPhen, A Diet 'Miracle,' Rose and Fell. New York Tmes.

Meadows, M. (2006, February). Centennial Edition of FDA Consumer - Promoting Safe and Effective Drugs for 100 Years. Retrieved January 14, 2018, from
https://www.fda.gov/AboutFDA/WhatWeDo/History/CentennialofFDA/CentennialEditionofFDAConsumer/ucm093787.htm

Mello, M. M., Studdert, D. M., & Brennan, T. A. (2009). Shifting Terrain in the Regulation of Off-Label Promotion of Pharmaceuticals. *New England Journal of Medicine,360*(15), 1557-1566. doi:10.1056/nejmhle0807695

Mundy, A. (2001). *Dispensing with the truth: the victims, the drug companies, and the dramatic story behind the battle over Fen-Phen*. New York: St. Martins Press.

NBC News (January 15, 2009). Eli Lilly settles Zyprexa lawsuit for $1.42 billion. (2009, January 15). Retrieved January 15, 2018, from http://www.nbcnews.com/id/28677805/ns/health-health_care/t/eli-lilly-settles-zyprexa-lawsuit-billion/
Associated Press

O'Reilly, J., & Dalal, A. (2003). Off-Label or out of Bounds? Prescriber and Marketer Liability for Unapproved Uses of FDA Approved Drugs. *Annals of Health Law,12*(2), 295-325. Retrieved January 14, 2018.

Rheingold, D. P. & Rheingold. B. D. (March 2001). Offense or Defense/Managing the Off-Label Use Claim. *TRIAL,52*, 52`-55.

Saul, S. (2005, February 17). Fen-Phen Case Lawyers Say They'll Reject Wyeth Offer. *New York Tmes.*

THOMPSON V. WESTERN STATES MEDICAL CENTER (01-344) 535 U. S. 357 (2002) 238 F.3d 1090, affirmed (April 29, 2002).
No. 01-344

US Department of Justice (January 2009). Eli Lilly and Company Agrees to Pay $1.415 Billion to Resolve Allegations of Off-label Promotion of Zyprexa. (n.d.). Retrieved January 15, 2018, from https://www.justice.gov/archive/opa/pr/2009/January/09-civ-038.html

Ventola, C. L. (August 2009). Off-Label Drug Information Regulation, Distribution, Evaluation, and Related Controversies. *Pharmacy and Therapeutics,34*(8), 428-440.

Washington Legal Foundation v. Friedman, 13 F. Supp. 2d 51 (D.D.C. 1998) (U.S. District Court for the District of Columbia July 30, 1998).
`
Weintraub, M., Sundaresan, P. R., Madan, M., Schuster, B., Balder, A., Lasagna, L., & Cox, C. (1992). Long-term weight control study I (weeks 0 to 34). *Clinical Pharmacology and Therapeutics,51*(5), 586-594. doi:10.1038/clpt.1992.69

Weintraub, M., Sundaresan, P. R., Schuster, B., Averbuch, M., Stein, E. C., Cox, C., & Byrne, L. (1992). Long-term weight control study IV (weeks 156 to

190). *Clinical Pharmacology and Therapeutics,51*(5), 608-614. doi:10.1038/clpt.1992.72

Wellman, P., & Maher, T. (1999). Synergistic interactions between Fenfluramine and Phentermine. *International Journal of Obesity,23*(7), 723-732. doi:10.1038/sj.ijo.0800920

Further Reading

Fang, F. C., Steen, R. G., & Casadevall, A. (2012). Misconduct accounts for the majority of retracted scientific publications. Proceedings of the National Academy of Sciences,109(42), 17028-17033. doi:10.1073/pnas.1212247109

Mello, M. M., Studdert, D. M., & Brennan, T. A. (2009). Shifting Terrain in the Regulation of Off-Label Promotion of Pharmaceuticals. *New England Journal of Medicine,360*(15), 1557-1566. doi:10.1056/nejmhle0807695

O'Reilly, J., & Dalal, A. (2003). Off-Label or out of Bounds? Prescriber and Marketer Liability for Unapproved Uses of FDA Approved Drugs. *Annals of Health Law,12*(2), 295-325. Retrieved January 14, 2018.

Conclusion

Medicine ... is an imperfect science, an enterprise of constantly changing knowledge, uncertain information, fallible individuals, and, at the same time, lives on the line. — Atul Gawande, *Complications*

Conclusion

In this book, we have examined failed visual perceptions, psychological biases, logical fallacies, misjudgments involving numbers, misinterpretation of tests, flawed or manipulated medical studies, and misunderstandings about medications.

Our journey has taken us across the academic countryside from medicine to jurisprudence, with stops along the way at psychology, logic, statistics, experimental design, and even conjuring.

The reasons for our journey are, of course, that we are not so rational as we would like to think, that we are blind to many of our own biases, and that we too often fail to allow for the unknown unknowns.

Other factors then compound these limitations. The imperative to publish or perish expands the volume of studies, sometimes to the detriment of their quality. The profit motive drives the introduction of expensive new drugs and medical devices, often no better than existing treatments. The desire to be seen as cutting edge drives the uncritical use of these new drugs and devices. The need to recoup high acquisition costs expands the unthinking use of new technology. The competition to be seen as advancing science often brings about only a *perception* of scientific advancement. Finally, the freedom of speech protection dubiously applied to pharmaceutical off-label claims threatens to undo hard-won, and often delayed, FDA public health protections.

We have, throughout the book, offered powerful countermeasures against failures of medical thinking. We offer now the challenge to implement these countermeasures in various venues.

In the university, it is time –
- To devote research to the investigation of medical decision making: how it *is* done, and how it *should be* done.
- To make better medical decision making part of medical education and continuing medical education.
- To adopt, adapt, and apply logic and statistics more rigorously to the medical curriculum, either integral with it or as prerequisite to it.

In the arena of public policy, it is time –
- To advocate for all trials to be registered and published in order to reduce the concealment of negative and inconclusive trials.

- To re-examine legislation on commercial free speech to prevent pharmaceutical industry circumvention of FDA public protections.
- To adopt, adapt, and apply more rigorously the *cognitive* safety measures developed and successfully employed by the aviation industry.

In clinical practice, it is time –
- To consult systematic reviews of large bodies of literature, instead of accepting as definitive a single journal article distributed by a "detail" person.
- To see medicine with a broader vision, passing beyond information's sometimes-unreliable content and, instead, more intensively examining information's quality, independence, and pertinence.
- To adopt, adapt, and apply the decision-making methods developed by psychologists and management researchers for other important areas of endeavor.

This book is a forceful call to action for educators, policy makers, and clinicians to apply this new dimension of better medical decision making to research, administration, and patient care. It is a forceful call to action for us to accept the challenge of responsibility from our patients, our peers, and ourselves. Above all, the book is a forceful call to action to think for ourselves, to maintain our intellectual independence, and to advocate for our patients in our practices, in the public media, and, especially, in the offices of our legislators.

Thomas Falasca, DO FACA FACPM
Erie, Pennsylvania, USA

Further Reading

Angell, M. (2004). The truth about the drug companies: how they deceive us and what to do about it. New York City, NY: Random House.

Barraclough, K. (2013). *Avoiding errors in general practice.* Chichester, West Sussex: Wiley-Blackwell.

Chabris, C. F., & Simons, D. J. (2012). *The invisible gorilla: and other ways our intuitions deceive us.* New York: MJF Books

Croskerry, P. (2002). Achieving Quality in Clinical Decision Making: Cognitive Strategies and Detection of Bias. *Academic Emergency Medicine, 9*(11), 1184-1204. doi:10.1197/aemj.9.11.1184

Darley, J. M., & Latane, B. (1968). Bystander intervention in emergencies: Diffusion of responsibility. Journal of Personality and Social Psychology,8(4, Pt.1), 377-383. doi:10.1037/h0025589

Drew, T., Võ, M. L. H., & Wolfe, J. M. (2013). The Invisible Gorilla Strikes Again: Sustained Inattentional Blindness in Expert Observers. *Psychological Science, 24*(9), 1848-1853. DOI: 10.1177/0956797613479386

Fang, F. C., Steen, R. G., & Casadevall, A. (2012). Misconduct accounts for the majority of retracted scientific publications. Proceedings of the National Academy of Sciences,109(42), 17028-17033. doi:10.1073/pnas.1212247109

Gigerenzer, G. (2015). *Risk savvy: how to make good decisions.* London: Penguin Books.

Gigerenzer, G. (2013). Better doctors, better patients, better decisions: envisioning health care 2020;. Cambridge, Mass.: MIT Press.

Gigerenzer, G., Gaissmaier, W., Kurz-Milcke, E., Schwartz, L., & Woloshin, S. (2008). Helping Doctors and Patients Make Sense of Health Statistics. Psychological Science in the Public Interest,8(2), 53-96.

Gigerenzer, G. (1996). The Psychology of Good Judgment. *Medical Decision Making,16*(3), 273-280. doi:10.1177/0272989x9601600312

Gilovich, T., Griffin, D., & Kahneman, D. (2005). Heuristics and biases: The psychology of intuitive judgment. Cambridge: Cambridge University Press.

Goldacre, B. (2010). Bad science: quacks, hacks and big pharma -- flacks --. New York: Faber and Faber.

Goldacre, B. (2014). Bad pharma: how drug companies mislead doctors and harm patients. New York: Faber & Faber, Inc., an affiliate of Farrar, Straus and Giroux.

Gøtzsche, P. C., Hróbjartsson, A., Johansen, H. K., Haahr, M. T., Altman, D. G., & Chan, A. (2006). Constraints on Publication Rights in Industry-Initiated Clinical Trials. Jama,295(14), 1641. doi:10.1001/jama.295.14.1645

Greenhalgh, T. (2014). *How to Read a Paper: The Basics of Evidence-based Medicine*. Wiley-Blackwell.

Groopman, J. E. (2010). *How doctors think*. Carlton North, Vic.: Scribe Publications.

Gurusamy, K. (2017, September 14). Interpretation of Forest Plots - Part 1. Lecture presented at Interpretation of Forest Plots - Part 1, London, UK. Lecture - University College London

Kahneman, D. (2015). *Thinking, fast and slow*. New York: Farrar, Straus and Giroux.

Kruger, J., & Dunning, D. (1999). Unskilled and unaware of it: How difficulties in recognizing one's own incompetence lead to inflated self-assessments. *Journal of Personality and Social Psychology, 77*(6), 1121-1134. doi:10.1037//0022-3514.77.6.1121

Macknik, S. L., Martinez-Conde, S., & Blakeslee, S. (2012). Sleights of mind: what the neuroscience of magic reveals about our brains. London: Profile.

Mello, M. M., Studdert, D. M., & Brennan, T. A. (2009). Shifting Terrain in the Regulation of Off-Label Promotion of Pharmaceuticals. *New England Journal of Medicine,360*(15), 1557-1566. doi:10.1056/nejmhle0807695

Milgram, S. (1963). Behavioral Study of obedience. *The Journal of Abnormal and Social Psychology,67*(4), 371-378. doi:10.1037/h0040525

Novella, S. (2012). Your deceptive mind: a scientific guide to critical thinking skills. Chantilly, VA: Teaching Company.

Novella, S., Gorski, D., & Crislip, M. (2013). Science-Based Medicine: Guide to Critical Thinking. Fort Lauderdale, FL: James Randi Educational Foundation. Kindle Edition

Novella, S. (2018). *The Skeptic's Guide to the Universe*. New York, NY: Grand Central Publishing.

O'Reilly, J., & Dalal, A. (2003). Off-Label or out of Bounds? Prescriber and Marketer Liability for Unapproved Uses of FDA Approved Drugs. *Annals of Health Law,12*(2), 295-325. Retrieved January 14, 2018.

Sedgwick, P. (2015, July 24). How to read a forest plot in a meta-analysis. Retrieved September 14, 2017, from http://www.bmj.com/content/351/bmj.h4028

Shermer, Michael. (2012). *The Believing Brain: From Ghosts and Gods to Politics and Conspiracies---How We Construct Beliefs and Reinforce Them as Truths. Henry Holt and Co.. Kindle Edition.*

Simel, D. L., Keitz, S. A., & Rennie, D. (2009). *The Rational clinical examination: evidence-based clinical diagnosis*. New York: McGraw-Hill Medical/JAMA & Archives Journals.
Simon, S. D. (2009). *Statistical evidence in medical trials: What do the data really tell us?*Oxford: Oxford University Press.

Song, F., Hooper, L., & Loke, Y. (2013). Publication bias: what is it? How do we measure it? How do we avoid it? Open Access Journal of Clinical Trials,71-81. doi:10.2147/oajct.s34419

Tramer, M. R., Reynolds, D. J., Moore, R. A., & Mcquay, H. J. (1997). Impact of covert duplicate publication on meta-analysis: a case study. Bmj,315(7109), 635-640. doi:10.1136/bmj.315.7109.635

Tversky, A., & Kahneman, D. (1974). Judgment under Uncertainty: Heuristics and Biases. *Science, 185*(4157), 1124-1131. doi:10.1126/science.185.4157.1124

University of Leicester. (2017, February 24). Controversial test could be leading to unnecessary open-heart operations. ScienceDaily. Retrieved September 18, 2017 from www.sciencedaily.com/releases/2017/02/170224092537.htm

Vishton, P. M. (2011). Understanding the Secrets of Human Perception. The Teaching Company - The Great Courses. doi:10.1037/e527652012-001

Welch, H. G. (2000). Are Increasing 5-Year Survival Rates Evidence of Success Against Cancer? *Jama,283*(22), 2975. doi:10.1001/jama.283.22.2975

Welch, H. G., Schwartz, L., & Woloshin, S. (2012). *Overdiagnosed: Making people sick in the pursuit of health*. New York: Random House.

Woloshin, S., Schwartz, L. M., & Welch, H. G. (2009). Know your chances: understanding health statistics. Berkeley: University of California Press

Index

Manning, 66, 69, 281
Marcus, 186, 187, 188, 190, 281
Marshall, 90, 93, 281
Massengill Company, 233
Matles test, 47
Mayo Lung Project, 185, 186, 187, 188, 190, 281, 283
McBride, 235
McCoy, 91
McKelvie, 193, 201, 286
Meadows, 231, 232, 240, 243, 254, 282
mean, 35, 89, 109, 113, 141, 146, 149, 150, 151, 153, 186, 199, 208, 209, 220, 222, 245, 246
measles, 42, 43, 171
measles-mumps-rubella, 42
medical decisions, 9, 10, 39, 49
medical interventions, 65
medical professional liability, 35, 63
medical tests, 9
medications, 10, 28, 61, 63, 66, 86, 99, 217, 231, 236, 237, 238, 243, 249, 250, 259
Medvedeva, 39, 50, 270
Mehta, 114, 120, 282
Mello, 50, 244, 249, 250, 252, 255, 256, 262, 270, 282
Memmert, 15, 22, 282
Merrell Company, 234, 235
mesothelioma, 145
meta-study, 195, 198
miasma, 125
Michelson, 134
Milgram, 5, 83, 84, 85, 92, 93, 262, 282
Mill, 135, 137, 282
Miller, 68, 223, 226, 269, 278, 282
Mintz, 234, 240, 282
misdirection, 14
Mitroff, 108, 111, 273
MMR, 42, 43, 50, 277
Molière, 130, 131, 283
Molloy, 220
Monty Hall Problem, 158, 159, 162, 278

Morley, 134
morphine, 72, 74, 133, 247
mortality rates, 186
motorcycle, 13, 19
Moyer, 182, 190, 283
Mozart effect, 193, 201, 269
multi-test panel, 152
Mundy, 244, 245, 255, 283
Murtagh, 48, 51, 283
Myers, 76, 77, 279

N

National Institute of Health, 182
natural frequency, 97, 157, 158, 159, 160, 161
necessary condition, 127, 168
negating the consequent, 124, 125, 168, 169
negligence, 67, 87, 131
NEJM, 198
New England Journal of Medicine, 51, 69, 93, 98, 105, 175, 179, 198, 208, 212, 226, 236, 238, 239, 245, 254, 255, 256, 262, 265, 269, 272, 275, 280, 281, 282, 287, 290, 292
Nexium, 130
nirvana Fallacy, 133, 135, 136
NNTT, 221
no-difference, 207, 208, 210, 211
non-responders, 194, 196
nonsteroidal anti-inflammatory drug, 248
normal curve, 5, 149
Novella, 42, 48, 49, 51, 52, 77, 114, 120, 127, 128, 198, 201, 202, 211, 212, 262, 284
novelty bias, 5, 67, 99, 100, 103
NSAID, 248
null hypothesis, 150
number needed to treat, 221, 225

O

O'Connor, 251
O'Reilly, 243, 248, 249, 252
Office of Research Integrity, 205
off-label advertising, 6, 243, 249

off-label reprints, 249
OJ Simpson Case, 126
olanzapine, 247
ondansetron, 195
open cholecystectomy, 196
open-access journals, 214
ophthalmologists, 87
optimum examination time, 111
orderly data collection, 48
Orlowski, 89, 93, 284
outcome measures, 197, 198, 200
overconfidence bias, 19, 53, 54, 55, 56, 57, 58, 67, 71

P

paclitaxel, 223, 225
Palacios-Huerta, 61, 69, 284
Palermo, 129, 132, 284
pancuronium, 27, 28
paroxetine, 199
patient identification, 28
patient pressure, 66
Paulos, 155, 162, 284
Pearson, 110, 111, 284
Pelé's shirt, 126
Pepcid, 26
perfect solution fallacy, 135
pericarditis, 114
per-protocol analysis, 195, 202
pertussis, 156
Pescetti, 135
Pfizer, 248
pharyngitis, 124, 131, 151
phentermine, 244, 245, 246
phlogiston, 125
Pillemer, 208, 212, 280
Piso's Consumption Cure, 231
Planck, 156, 184
planning bias, 71, 246
planning fallacy, 71, 72, 73
Pondimin, 244, 245
poor replicability, 193
popitis, 102
Popper, 151, 154, 285
post hoc, 5, 123, 125, 126
Potchen, 18, 22, 56, 57, 59, 285

Prasad, 46, 47, 91, 92, 265
Prayle, 213, 215, 285
prehypertension, 35
Prilosec, 130
problems with surveys, 64
projecting one year into the future, 58
Pronin, 53, 54, 59, 285
Prontosil, 233
prostate specific antigen, 172, 182
PSA, 172, 173, 182, 184, 189, 277, 285
psychological bias, 33, 85
Public Library of Science, 214, 215, 274
Publication Bias, 6, 207, 208, 210, 212, 279, 284
PubMed, 203, 249
pulmonary artery catheterization, 62
pulmonary edema, 17, 18, 19, 21
pulmonary emboli, 17
Purcell, 142

Q

quality-of-life, 224
Quattrocchi, 110, 112, 285
quinine, 234

R

Radiothor, 233
random sample, 141, 150
randomization, 194, 196
randomized clinical trial, 207, 223, 226, 277
randomness, 5, 141, 142, 144
Rauscher, 193, 285
Ray, 222, 227, 286
RCT, 207, 222
reasonable and prudent, 88, 92
reductionism, 44
Redux, 244, 245
reference class forecasting, 73
reference range, 150, 151, 152, 153
reference to the population base-rate, 57
reframe the information, 97

Made in the USA
Monee, IL
25 March 2022

93566530R00151